MW01630374

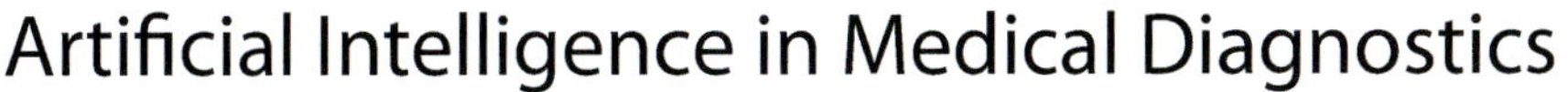

Artificial Intelligence in Medical Diagnostics

Takanobu Hirosawa

Artificial Intelligence in Medical Diagnostics

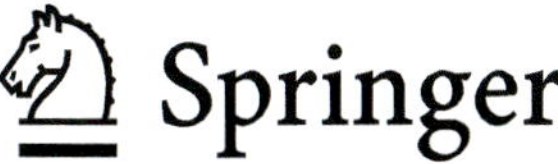

Takanobu Hirosawa
Department of Diagnostic and Generalist Medicine
Dokkyo Medical University
Simotsuga-gun, Tochigi, Japan

ISBN 978-981-95-4337-3 ISBN 978-981-95-4338-0 (eBook)
https://doi.org/10.1007/978-981-95-4338-0

This Springer imprint is published by the registered company Springer Nature Singapore Pte Ltd.
The registered company address is: 152 Beach Road, #21-01/04 Gateway East, Singapore 189721, Singapore

Introduction

This book serves as a foundational guide to bridge the knowledge gap between the rapidly advancing field of artificial intelligence and the established practices of medical diagnostics, designed with a dual purpose: to introduce and to bridge the gap between two distinct but increasingly interconnected fields. Whether you are a healthcare professional stepping into the transformative world of artificial intelligence for the first time or an artificial intelligence developer seeking deeper insights into medical contexts, this book offers a comprehensive and accessible resource.

For healthcare professionals, the rapidly evolving landscape of artificial intelligence can be exciting. This book simplifies the complex world of artificial intelligence, presenting key concepts and applications in a manner that avoids overwhelming technical jargon and mathematical intricacies. For artificial intelligence developers, this book emphasizes the importance of understanding the realities of clinical practices, workflows, and patient care, ensuring that their technological innovations align with the practical needs and ethical responsibilities of the healthcare domain.

At its core, this book explores the transformative potential of artificial intelligence to revolutionize diagnostic medicine. By automating complex analyses, uncovering subtle patterns in data, and offering new levels of precision and efficiency, artificial intelligence holds the promise of enhancing diagnostic accuracy and patient outcomes. However, this journey is not without challenges and limitations. To navigate this new frontier, healthcare professionals and artificial intelligence developers must also understand the limitations and risks associated with artificial intelligence, including issues like data bias, lack of transparency, and ethical dilemmas.

While this book will not teach you how to develop artificial intelligence for medical diagnostics, it will provide you with the knowledge necessary to understand, evaluate, and collaborate with artificial intelligence systems effectively. For healthcare professionals, this means learning how to integrate artificial intelligence tools into medicine, especially medical diagnosis. For artificial intelligence developers, this book provides a valuable lens into the medical environment, fostering an understanding of the stakes and sensitivities involved in patient care. The goal is to promote collaboration between these two groups, cultivating a hybrid intelligence that combines human expertise and artificial intelligence capabilities to deliver more accurate, efficient, and patient-centered diagnostics.

Finally, it is essential to recognize the dynamic and ever-changing nature of digital health technologies, particularly artificial intelligence. Alongside climate change, artificial intelligence represents one of the most significant changes humanity faces today. Its influence extends deeply into how we live, work, communicate, and provide care, particularly in critical sectors such as health care. Understanding and adapting to these transformative forces is essential for building a future that is both technologically advanced and ethically grounded. While this book provides a robust foundation, it is by no means an endpoint. Both healthcare professionals and artificial intelligence developers must commit to continuous learning, staying informed about the latest research, advancements, and best practices in their respective fields. Only through an ongoing commitment to growth and collaboration can the transformative potential of artificial intelligence in medical diagnostics be fully realized and responsibly harnessed for the benefit of patients and society.

Acknowledgments

Thank you to my family for always supporting me. Thank you, Dr. Yukinori Harada, for reviewing this book throughout this process and encouraging me to publish this book. Much appreciation to faculty and mentors at the Department of Diagnostic and Generalist Medicine in Dokkyo Medical University for always lending a helpful ear and providing constructive feedback.

Contents

Introduction to Medical Diagnosis

1

Abstract

This first chapter explores the foundational principles, complexities, and challenges of medical diagnosis, highlighting its central role in clinical care. Accurate and timely diagnosis is essential for effective management, prevention, and improved patient outcomes. This chapter emphasizes the dynamic and iterative nature of the diagnostic process, which involves integrating diverse clinical data, hypothesis testing, and evidence-based reasoning. The chapter begins by defining medical diagnosis and discussing its importance in individual patient care and public health. The discussion turns to the traditional cognitive science underpinning medical diagnosis, emphasizing the dual processes of heuristic (System 1) and analytic (System 2) reasoning. Bayesian theory is introduced as a critical framework for refining diagnostic probabilities based on evolving clinical information. Cognitive biases that challenge diagnostic accuracy, such as anchoring, availability, and confirmation biases, are examined and paralleled with data biases in artificial intelligence, highlighting shared challenges in human and machine-assisted diagnostics. Key diagnostic performance metrics, involving sensitivity, specificity, and likelihood ratio, are detailed. The trade-offs inherent in these metrics are discussed in the context of clinical decision-making. Modern diagnostic complexities are addressed, alongside the risks of diagnostic errors, overdiagnosis, and underdiagnosis. Strategies to achieve diagnostic excellence are outlined, emphasizing a multidisciplinary, team-based approach, clinical decision support systems, and system-level improvements. The chapter concludes organizations' initiatives to promote diagnostic excellence globally.

Keywords

Medical diagnosis · Diagnostic process · Cognitive biases · Clinical reasoning · Diagnostic performance · Overdiagnosis · Underdiagnosis · Diagnostic excellence

T. Hirosawa, *Artificial Intelligence in Medical Diagnostics*,
https://doi.org/10.1007/978-981-95-4338-0_1

1.1 Medical Diagnosis

Medical diagnosis lies at the center of clinical practice, guiding health-care professionals in determining the most appropriate treatment pathways for their patients. Accurate and timely diagnosis is essential for effective medical management, disease prevention, and the improvement of patient outcomes. Despite its importance, diagnostic accuracy remains challenging due to the complexity and volume of clinical information that must be analyzed, interpreted, and integrated into clinical decisions.

In modern health care, the available data for diagnosis has dramatically increased. This data includes detailed patients' medical histories, comprehensive physical examinations, extensive diagnostic imaging, and advanced laboratory investigations. The exponential growth in diagnostic information elevates cognitive load on health-care professionals, potentially leading to diagnostic errors. Addressing this challenge necessitates innovative tools and technological advancements to improve diagnostic accuracy and efficiency. This chapter introduces medical diagnosis, emphasizes its critical roles, elucidates its inherent complexities, and identifies the challenges to achieving diagnostic excellence.

1.1.1 What Is Medical Diagnosis?

Medical diagnosis is far more than labeling a patient's condition. Instead, it represents a dynamic and iterative process that integrates multiple sources of clinical information to accurately identify the nature and underlying causes of patient symptoms [1]. The diagnostic process includes comprehensive history taking, systematic patient observation, hypothesis formulation, rigorous clinical reasoning, and testing hypotheses through targeted investigations, underpinned by evidence-based medical principles.

Diagnosis is not a static, singular event. It continuously evolves as additional clinical information becomes available through ongoing patient interaction, diagnostic investigations, and clinical courses. This iterative nature requires health-care professionals to adapt and refine their diagnostic hypotheses continually. Another essential aspect of the diagnostic process is the integration of clinical guidelines and the application of current research findings. Clinical guidelines, developed by the best available evidence, provide structured recommendations that help health-care professionals standardize care and reduce variability in diagnosis. Additionally, the continuous emergence of new research findings means health-care professionals must regularly update their diagnostic approaches to reflect the advanced medical knowledge.

Successful diagnosis facilitates targeted treatment, prognosis prediction, and patient-centered care, engaging patients and their families in shared decision-making processes. Moreover, medical diagnosis plays a critical role in public health by identifying disease trends, monitoring early detection of outbreaks, and informing preventative strategies.

1.1.2 Importance of Medical Diagnosis

Medical diagnosis is foundational to the effective delivery of patient care and the overall functionality of health-care systems. A timely and accurate diagnosis optimizes clinical outcomes by ensuring prompt, appropriate treatment, minimizing unnecessary interventions, and reducing associated health care costs. Furthermore, diagnosis extends beyond clinical significance, carrying substantial psychological and social importance for patients. Obtaining a precise diagnosis provides individuals with clarity regarding their health status, reduces anxiety associated with uncertainty, and empowers them with the knowledge necessary to engage in informed decision-making about their health-care journey [2].

1.2 Diagnostic Process

The diagnostic process is the cornerstone of medical practice. The process is inherently complex, involving not only the collection and interpretation of clinical data but also the influence of human cognition, contextual factors, and decision-making frameworks. Understanding how diagnoses are formed, and the potential pitfalls that can compromise accuracy, is critical for improving patient outcomes.

1.2.1 Cognitive Science of Diagnosis

From cognitive science frameworks, the diagnostic process is traditionally conceptualized within two primary frameworks: intuitive reasoning (System 1) and analytic reasoning (System 2) [3]. Effective diagnosis often involves a dynamic interplay between both systems—using System 1 for routine cases and engaging System 2 for complex or unusual ones. These cognitive systems describe distinct but complementary approaches to health-care professionals utilizing clinical decision-making.

Intuitive reasoning, referred to as heuristic reasoning or System 1 thinking, characterized by rapid, intuitive judgments. It is heavily based on pattern recognition by health-care professionals with clinical experience. Experienced health-care professionals often rely on intuitive reasoning, quickly identifying familiar patterns of symptoms, which enables swift clinical decision-making in typical cases. However, reliance on intuitive reasoning, referred to as a cognitive shortcut, increases vulnerability to cognitive biases, potentially impacting diagnostic accuracy. Common cognitive biases associated with System 1 include anchoring, overreliance on initial impressions or information, and availability bias, favoring diagnoses that readily come to mind due to recent experience or emotional salience. These cognitive pitfalls and their implications are further detailed in Sect. 1.2.2.

Analytic reasoning, or System 2 thinking, contrasts with the heuristic approach by involving conscious and structured thought processes. Health-care professionals employing analytic reasoning methodically evaluate clinical data, logically test diagnostic hypotheses, and rigorously appraise evidence. While this systematic and reflective approach is inherently slower and requires greater cognitive effort, it serves to reduce, though not eliminate, susceptibility to certain cognitive biases (e.g., confirmation bias, anchoring) [4, 5]. It is especially advantageous in situations characterized by complexity, diagnostic uncertainty, or atypical presentations that do not align well with familiar clinical patterns.

Bayesian theory serves as an essential mathematical and conceptual framework underlying clinical reasoning processes, integrating the concepts inherent in both System 1 and System 2 reasoning. Bayesian reasoning provides a structured method for adjusting diagnostic probabilities considering newly acquired clinical information. Health-care professionals start by establishing pretest probability, which represents their initial estimate of the likelihood of a condition based on initial assessments, including patient history and epidemiological context. As further diagnostic evidence emerges—such as physical examination findings, laboratory test outcomes, or imaging studies—health-care professionals revise this probability to determine a more precise posttest probability. This dynamic, iterative approach helps health-care professionals systematically refine their diagnoses, optimizing clinical decisions through continuous incorporation of evidence. Bayesian reasoning thus stands as a cornerstone in contemporary diagnostic science, promoting evidence-based practices that enhance diagnostic accuracy and patient outcomes.

1.2.2 Bias in Diagnostic Process

Cognitive biases are systematic, predictable errors in reasoning that significantly impact judgment and decision-making processes [1]. These biases influence health-care professionals' clinical reasoning, potentially leading to diagnostic errors, delayed treatment initiation, compromised patient outcomes, and increased health-care costs. Common cognitive biases in medical diagnosis include anchoring bias, availability bias, affective bias, and confirmation bias.

- Anchoring Bias: Anchoring bias refers to the tendency of health-care professionals to rely excessively on their initial impressions, diagnoses, or information obtained early. For example, a health-care professional might initially diagnose a patient with viral pharyngitis based on common presenting symptoms such as fever and sore throat. This initial assessment might cause the professionals to inadvertently overlook critical signs indicative of more serious conditions, such as drooling of saliva or muffled voice indicating acute epiglottitis [6]. Health-care professionals may rely on outputs provided by artificial intelligence systems, resulting in diagnostic complacency and reduced scrutiny of conflicting clinical information.
- Availability Bias: Availability bias describes health-care professionals' propensity to diagnose diseases that come most readily to mind often influenced by recent clinical experience or highly memorable cases. This cognitive shortcut occurs when frequent or emotionally impactful clinical encounters

disproportionately influence diagnostic judgment. For instance, during a period of increased seasonal influenza cases, a primary care physician may easily attribute a patient's respiratory symptoms to seasonal influenza, missing a diagnosis of bacterial pneumonia, thus delaying appropriate treatment. This bias emphasizes the critical need for health-care professionals to evaluate each clinical case independently, rather than relying on the familiar patterns.
- Affective Bias: Affective bias arises when health-care professionals' personal emotions, attitudes, or implicit biases influence decision-making processes, often subconsciously. Emotional reactions or implicit prejudices may lead health-care professionals to either downplay or exaggerate symptoms and clinical findings, affecting their clinical judgments and decisions. For example, implicit biases might lead a health-care professional to underestimate or dismiss the significance of fatigue reported by younger patients, potentially resulting in missed diagnoses such as hypothyroidism or iron deficiency anemia. Addressing affective biases necessitates enhancing health-care professionals' awareness of implicit bias, adopting structured decision-making frameworks, and promoting equitable care to minimize disparities in clinical outcomes.
- Confirmation Bias: Confirmation bias represents health-care professionals' tendency to selectively seek, prioritize, or interpret clinical information that confirms their initial diagnostic hypotheses while undervaluing or disregarding conflicting evidence. Health-care professionals exhibiting confirmation bias might focus extensively on information that reinforces their initial diagnostic impression, thereby limiting their ability to objectively consider alternative diagnoses. For example, a health-care professional suspecting congestive heart failure might prioritize supportive clinical findings such as shortness of breath and pulmonary vascular congestion in chest radiograph, yet disregard or inadequately consider no leg edema and low B-type natriuretic peptide levels, which could indicate another underlying condition [7]. Such selective information processing significantly hampers accurate clinical decision-making, leading to inappropriate treatments and patient harm.

These cognitive biases substantially contribute to diagnostic errors, delayed treatment, and poor patient outcomes. Mitigating cognitive biases requires deliberate cultivation of self-awareness, continuous education, and implementation of structured clinical protocols and promoting practices that encourage systematic reflection and critical analysis [8, 9]. Collectively, these strategies foster enhanced clinical judgement, diagnostic accuracy, and improved patient safety and health outcomes.

1.2.3 Comparing Cognitive Bias, Data Bias, and Algorithmic Bias in Artificial Intelligence

Bias represents a significant shared concern in both human diagnostic processes and artificial intelligence systems. The term "bias" itself has intersectional implications across medicine and artificial intelligence, a topic explored in detail within Chap. 4.

Further comparative analysis between biases inherent in human diagnostic processes and those found within artificial intelligence training datasets, as well as biases introduced by algorithmic structures themselves, is discussed comprehensively in Chap. 10.

Human diagnostic bias typically originates from cognitive processes. Such cognitive biases include heuristic shortcuts and emotional influences, all of which can distort diagnostic accuracy and reliability. Heuristic shortcuts, although efficient, may cause health-care professionals to overly rely on familiar patterns or memorable cases, potentially leading to incorrect diagnoses. Cognitive biases highlight the subjective nature of human decision-making, despite extensive professional training.

Conversely, biases within artificial intelligence typically stem from two principal sources: data utilized in model training processes, termed "data bias," and structural limitations of the algorithms themselves, termed "algorithmic bias." Data bias arises from limitations in the quality, representativeness, and comprehensiveness of datasets used to train artificial intelligence models. For example, an artificial intelligence diagnostic model trained primarily on datasets inadequately representing specific demographics or conditions will likely exhibit reduced diagnostic accuracy when applied to underrepresented populations. Such biases can perpetuate existing health-care inequities and disproportionately disadvantage marginalized groups [10].

Algorithmic bias arises independently of data issues, emerging instead from the inherent characteristics and assumptions embedded within the artificial intelligence algorithms. These biases can be introduced through overly simplistic modeling assumptions, inappropriate selection of model parameters, or optimization procedures favoring certain outcomes unintentionally. Such structural biases may lead to systematically skewed diagnostic predictions, even when the training data are unbiased and comprehensive [11].

All these forms—diagnostic bias in humans, data bias in artificial intelligence, and algorithmic bias—compromise the integrity and reliability of medical diagnostics. This integrated perspective highlights the urgency of developing robust detection and mitigation strategies. Subsequent chapters explore advanced methodologies and frameworks designed to identify and mitigate biases in artificial intelligence systems. Emphasis will be placed on highlighting similarity and difference between human and artificial diagnostic reasoning, providing a foundation for comprehensive bias mitigation strategies in health-care.

1.3 Diagnostic Performance

Diagnostic performance metrics are essential for evaluating the effectiveness and reliability of diagnostic processes. They provide insights into the trade-offs between detecting true cases of a disease and avoiding false results. Understanding these metrics is crucial for health-care professionals to interpret test results and optimize decision-making.

1.3.1 Confusion Matrix

The confusion matrix is a key tool for assessing the performance of diagnostic processes, as shown in Table 1.1. It categorizes test results into four distinct groups based on actual and predicted outcomes:

- True Positive (TP): Correctly predicted positive cases. For example, a patient with pneumonia correctly identified by a chest X-ray as having the disease
- False Negative (FN): Incorrectly predicted negative cases (Type II error, or a "miss"). For instance, failing to detect pneumonia in a patient who has the condition
- False Positive (FP): Incorrectly predicted positive cases (Type I error, or a "false alarm"). For example, diagnosing pneumonia in a patient who does not have the condition
- True Negative (TN): Correctly predicted negative cases. For instance, a healthy individual correctly identified as not having pneumonia

1.3.2 Accuracy, Sensitivity, and Specificity

The relationship between sensitivity and specificity is often a trade-off; increasing one often decreases the other. Health-care professionals must decide which metric to prioritize based on the clinical scenario. In real-world medicine, achieving both 100% sensitivity and specificity is extremely rare.

- Accuracy: The ratio between the correctly classified cases and the total number of cases
- Sensitivity also known as recall: The ability of a diagnostic test to correctly identify individuals with a condition (true positive ratio)
- Specificity: The ability of a test to correctly identify individuals without the condition (true negative ratio)

1.3.3 Positive Likelihood Ratio (PLR), Negative Likelihood Ratio (NLR), and F1 Score

Likelihood ratios provide a powerful way to interpret diagnostic tests because they are independent of disease prevalence and link directly to how test results change a pretest probability into a posttest probability.

Table 1.1 Confusion matrix

	Predicted positive	Predicted negative
Actual positive	True positive (TP)	False negative (FN, type II error or "miss")
Actual negative	False positive (FP, type I error or "false alarm")	True negative (TN)

- PLR (Positive Likelihood Ratio): Indicates how much more likely a positive test result is to be found in someone with the disease compared to someone without it. A higher PLR strengthens the evidence for the presence of disease. For example, the presence of an S3 heart sound has been shown to yield a high PLR for congestive heart failure in adults presenting with dyspnea to the emergency department [12].
- NLR (Negative Likelihood Ratio): Indicates how much less likely a negative test result is to be found in someone with the disease compared to someone without it. A lower NLR strengthens the evidence for ruling out disease. For instance, a negative d-dimer test in a low-risk patient results in a very low NLR, making pulmonary embolism highly unlikely [13].
- F1 score: F1 score combines precision and recall into a single metric to provide a balanced measure, especially in cases where there is an uneven class distribution (e.g., rare diseases). While the F1 score is common in the artificial intelligence domain [14], it is less frequently used in medical diagnostics. This is because other metrics, such as sensitivity and specificity, are considered more appropriate for evaluating medical diagnostic tools, especially when assessing risk prediction [15, 16]. Medical diagnostics often place different weights on false positives versus false negatives (e.g., a false negative for malignancy is often considered far more dangerous than a false positive), whereas the F1 score treats them with equal importance via the harmonic mean.

1.3.4 ROC Curve and AUC

- Receiver Operating Characteristic (ROC) Curve: Receiver Operating Characteristic (ROC) Curve: A graphical representation of a diagnostic test's performance across different decision thresholds. It plots the true positive rate (sensitivity) against the false positive rate (1 − specificity).
- AUC (Area Under Curve): The AUC quantifies the overall performance of a test, with a value closer to 1 indicating high accuracy. For example, a diagnostic imaging technique with an AUC of 0.95 is considered highly effective at differentiating diseases from healthy individuals.

1.3.5 Odds, Risk, and Odds Ratio

- Odds: Odds represent the ratio of the probability of an event occurring to it not occurring. For example, if 20 out of 100 patients develop a complication, the odds are 20:80 or 1:4.
- Risk: Risk is the probability of an event occurring. For the same example, the risk is 20/100 = 20%.
- Odds Ratio (OR): The odds ratio compares the odds of an event occurring in one group to the odds of it occurring in another group. For instance, if a new medication reduces the odds of developing a condition by 50%, the OR is 0.5. ORs are frequently used in case-control studies to evaluate risk factors [17].

1.3.6 Number Needed to Treat (NNT) and Number Needed to Harm (NNH)

- NNT: The NNT is the number of patients who need to receive a specific treatment to prevent one adverse event or achieve one beneficial outcome [18]. For example, if an anticoagulant prevents one stroke for every 25 patients treated, the NNT is 25. Lower NNT values indicate more effective interventions.
- NNH: The NNH is the number of patients who need to receive treatment for one person to experience an adverse effect [19]. For instance, if a medication causes significant bleeding in 1 out of 100 patients, the NNH is 100. Higher NNH values indicate safer treatments.

Health-care professionals must balance these metrics to optimize care. For example:

- A test with high sensitivity but low specificity might be preferred for initial screening to ensure no cases are missed, as seen in annual health check-up.
- Conversely, a confirmatory test might prioritize specificity to reduce false positives, as in cancer diagnosis.

By combining metrics like PLR, NLR, ROC curves, and AUC with practical measures such as NNT and NNH, health-care professionals can make informed decisions about the value and applicability of diagnostic tests in specific patient populations [20–22]. In the context of artificial intelligence, precision, recall, and F1 score are valuable tools for evaluating classification models [14]. Summary of the diagnostic metrics are shown in Table 1.2.

Table 1.2 Summary of the diagnostic metrics

Metric	Definition	Formula
Accuracy	Ratio between the correctly classified cases and the total number of cases	$\frac{\text{True Positives} + \text{True Negatives}}{\text{True Positive} + \text{False Positives} + \text{True Negatives} + \text{False Negatives}}$
Sensitivity (Recall)	Ability of a test to correctly identify individuals with the condition (true positive rate)	$\frac{\text{True Positives}}{\text{True Positives} + \text{False Negatives}}$
Specificity	Ability of a test to correctly identify individuals without the condition (true negative rate)	$\frac{\text{True Negatives}}{\text{True Negatives} + \text{False Positives}}$
Positive Likelihood Ratio (PLR)	How much more likely a positive test result is in patients with the disease compared to those without	$\frac{\text{Sensitivity}}{(1 - \text{Specificity})}$
Negative Likelihood Ratio (NLR)	How much less likely a negative test results is in patients with the disease compared to those without	$\frac{(1 - \text{Sensitivity})}{\text{Specificity}}$
*F*1 Score	Harmonic means of precision and recall, balancing false positives and false negatives	$2 \times \frac{\text{Precision} \times \text{Recall}}{\text{Precision} + \text{Recall}}$
ROC (Receiver Operating Characteristic) Curve	Graph showing sensitivity vs. (1 − specificity) at various thresholds	Plot of $\text{Sensitivity} = \frac{\text{True Positives}}{\text{True Positives} + \text{False Negatives}}$ vs. $1 - \text{Specificity} = \frac{\text{False Positives}}{\text{True Negatives} + \text{False Positives}}$

AUC (Area Under the Curve)	Summary of ROC curve performance; closer to 1 indicates better diagnostic accuracy	$\int_0^1 \text{ROC}(t)\,dt$ (integral of true positive rate over false positive rate) or Computed numerically using trapezoidal rules from ROC points
Risk	Probability of an event occurring.	$\frac{\text{Number of Events}}{\text{Total Population}}$
Odds	Ratio of the probability of an event occurring to it not occurring	$\frac{\text{Probability of Event}}{1-\text{Probability of Event}}$
Odds Ratio (OR)	Compares odds of an event between two groups	$\frac{\text{Odds in Group A}}{\text{Odds in Group B}}$
NNT (Number Needed to Treat)	Number of patients who need to be treated to prevent one adverse event or achieve one benefit	$\frac{1}{\text{Absolute Risk Reduction}}$
NNH (Number Needed to Harm)	Number of patients who need to be treated for one to experience an adverse effect	$\frac{1}{\text{Attributable Risk}}$

1.4 The Complexities of Modern Diagnosis

Modern diagnostics face increasing complexity due to technological advancements, an expanding array of diagnostic options, and the growing burden of health-care data. These factors introduce risks such as diagnostic errors, overdiagnosis, and underdiagnosis.

1.4.1 Diagnostic Errors

The report "To Err Is Human: Building a Safer Health System" by the Institute of Medicine highlighted the prevalence and consequences of diagnostic errors in 2000. The report concluded that the health-care system often falls short of optimal safety standards [23]. In 2015, the National Academy of Medicine offered a widely cited definition of diagnostic error as "the failure to (a) establish an accurate and timely explanation of *the patient's* health problem(s) or (b) communicate that explanation to *the patient*" [1]. This definition highlights the dual importance of both reaching the correct diagnosis and effectively conveying it to patients.

Diagnostic errors encompass a range of failures that can compromise patient outcomes. These errors can occur at various stages of the diagnostic process and include the following:

- Error or Delay in Diagnosis: A missed or delayed diagnosis can result in the progression of a disease and missed opportunities for early intervention. For example, failing to recognize the early signs of a stroke can lead to severe complications.
- Failure to Employ Indicated Tests: Omitting appropriate diagnostic tests, such as imaging or laboratory analyses, may leave critical information undiscovered, resulting in misdiagnosis.
- Use of Outmoded Tests or Therapy: Relying on outdated diagnostic techniques or treatments may lead to suboptimal care and missed opportunities for newer, more effective interventions.
- Failure to Act on Results of Monitoring or Testing: Ignoring or misinterpreting test results, such as abnormal lab findings or imaging studies, can result in missed diagnoses or delayed treatment.

These errors highlight the complexity of modern diagnosis, which requires health-care professionals to manage a vast array of clinical data while navigating systemic and cognitive challenges [23]. Contributing factors include cognitive biases, insufficient data, communication failures, and system-level inefficiencies.

1.4.2 Overdiagnosis Versus Underdiagnosis

Overdiagnosis is defined as when a condition is diagnosed that is unlikely to affect the individual's health or lead to harm. A common example is the detection of slow-growing cancers that might never cause symptoms during a patient's lifetime. Overdiagnosis can lead to unnecessary treatment, increased anxiety, and wasted resources [24]. In contrast, underdiagnosis refers to the failure to identify a condition in a timely manner. This can result in delayed treatment and worse outcomes, particularly in cases of rapidly progressing diseases [25].

1.4.3 Diagnostic Excellence

Beyond diagnostic error, diagnostic excellence includes the six dimensions of quality: care that is safe, effective, patient-centered, timely, efficient, and equitable [26]. This requires a combination of skilled clinical reasoning, effective use of diagnostic tools, and robust health-care systems. Diagnostic excellence is also closely tied to emphasizing clear communication, shared decision-making, and respect for patient preferences. Achieving diagnostic excellence may involve a balance among such competing dimensions [27].

Patient-centered diagnostic excellence extends beyond clinical accuracy to embrace a comprehensive approach that includes the patient's perspective. This approach involves valuing the patient's knowledge alongside the health-care professional's insights. It emphasizes ensuring long-term follow-up with attention to the patient's reports. Maintaining a balanced approach to diagnostic evaluations helps avoid over- or under-investigation. Enhancing the interpretability of diagnostic information for the patient is crucial. Finally, aligning medical language with the patient's understanding enhances a shared framework of care [28].

1.5 Challenge to Diagnostic Excellence

Achieving diagnostic excellence is a multifaceted challenge that requires addressing individual, team-based, and systemic factors [29].

1.5.1 Team-Based Approach

Diagnosis is increasingly recognized as a collaborative effort involving health-care professionals, patients, and their families. By fostering effective communication and teamwork, diagnostic teams can pool their expertise, reduce cognitive biases, and ensure a more comprehensive evaluation of complex cases. Team-based approaches are particularly valuable in multidisciplinary settings, where specialists contribute diverse perspectives to the diagnostic process.

1.5.2 Clinical Decision Support Systems

Advances in technology, particularly in clinical decision support systems, have the potential to transform the diagnostic landscape. Clinical decision support systems leverage algorithms, machine learning, and evidence-based guidelines to assist health-care professionals in generating differential diagnoses, interpreting test results, and identifying potential errors. By integrating these systems into clinical workflows, health-care professionals can enhance diagnostic accuracy and efficiency while reducing variability in care. The overview of clinical decision support systems is described in Chap. 3.

1.5.3 System-Level Challenges

At the system level, barriers to diagnostic excellence include inadequate training, fragmented communication, and limited access to resources. Addressing these challenges requires investment in education, infrastructure, and quality improvement initiatives [30]. Additionally, fostering a culture of safety and accountability can help health-care organizations identify and address diagnostic errors proactively.

1.6 Health Organizations and Diagnostic Excellence

Diagnostic excellence has increasingly become a global health priority. The following sections highlight the contributions of key institutions driving diagnostic excellence worldwide.

1.6.1 World Health Organization and Diagnostic Excellence

The World Health Organization's (WHO) has recognized the critical importance of accurate and timely diagnosis as a cornerstone of effective health-care. The 2024 World Patient Safety Day is a landmark initiative focusing on improving diagnosis. Key objectives of the WHO's diagnostic excellence initiatives include raising awareness among health-care professionals, patients, and policymakers about the importance of accurate and timely diagnosis as a critical component of patient safety. The WHO's efforts highlight the profound impact of diagnosis not only on individual patient outcomes but also on broader public health metrics. The WHO supports and promotes diagnostic excellence through various activities focused on:

- Raising Awareness: Increasing awareness among stakeholders (health-care professionals, patients, policymakers) about the critical role of accurate diagnosis
- Fostering Collaboration and Equity: Promoting collaboration among health-care providers, patients, and families, with a specific emphasis on addressing health equity and reaching underserved populations
- Leveraging Technology: Utilizing technology to improve diagnostic processes, particularly in resource-constrained settings
- Global Data and Benchmarking: Using global data and benchmarking to understand diagnostic errors and develop evidence-based strategies for improvement [31]

1.6.2 Centers for Disease Control and Prevention and Diagnostic Excellence

The Centers for Disease Control and Prevention has developed "Core Elements to promote diagnostic excellence" [32], a framework that guides hospitals and health-care systems in improving diagnostic practices [33]. Key aspects of this framework include the following:

- Structured workflows for gathering and analyzing clinical data
- Ongoing training for health-care professionals to enhance diagnostic reasoning and reduce cognitive biases
- Integration of technology, such as clinical decision support systems, to support accurate diagnosis

In conclusion, this chapter has highlighted the centrality of medical diagnosis in clinical practice and public health. Accurate diagnosis is the foundation upon which effective treatment, prevention, and patient-centered care are built. However, achieving diagnostic excellence is fraught with challenges, including cognitive biases, increasing data complexity, and systemic inefficiencies.

Ultimately, achieving diagnostic excellence requires a collective effort from health-care professionals, patients, policymakers, and global health organizations. The journey toward diagnostic excellence is ongoing. The next chapter will build on this foundation by exploring the historical evolution of diagnostic techniques, setting the stage for understanding how artificial intelligence and technological innovations are transforming the diagnostic landscape.

References

1. Balogh EP, Miller BT, Ball JR. Improving diagnosis in health care. Washington, DC: National Academies Press; 2015.
2. Jeske M, James J, Joyce K. Diagnosis and the practices of patienthood: how diagnostic journeys shape illness experiences. Sociol Health Illn. 2024;46(S1):225–41.

3. Croskerry P. A universal model of diagnostic reasoning. Acad Med. 2009;84(8):1022–8.
4. Webster CS, Taylor S, Weller JM. Cognitive biases in diagnosis and decision making during anaesthesia and intensive care. BJA Educ. 2021;21(11):420–5.
5. Norman GR, Monteiro SD, Sherbino J, Ilgen JS, Schmidt HG, Mamede S. The causes of errors in clinical reasoning: cognitive biases, knowledge deficits, and dual process thinking. Acad Med. 2017;92(1):23–30.
6. Glynn F, Fenton JE. Diagnosis and management of supraglottitis (Epiglottitis). Curr Infect Dis Rep. 2008;10(3):200–4.
7. Mull N, Reilly JB, Myers JS. An elderly woman with 'heart failure': cognitive biases and diagnostic error. Cleve Clin J Med. 2015;82(11):745–53.
8. Hershberger PJ, Markert RJ, Part HM, Cohen SM, Finger WW. Understanding and addressing cognitive bias in medical education. Adv Health Sci Educ Theory Pract. 1996;1(3):221–6.
9. Kramer HS, Drews FA. Checking the lists: a systematic review of electronic checklist use in health care. J Biomed Inform. 2017;71:S6–S12.
10. Challen R, Denny J, Pitt M, Gompels L, Edwards T, Tsaneva-Atanasova K. Artificial intelligence, bias and clinical safety. BMJ Qual Saf. 2019;28(3):231–7.
11. Abràmoff MD, Tarver ME, Loyo-Berrios N, Trujillo S, Char D, Obermeyer Z, et al. Considerations for addressing bias in artificial intelligence for health equity. NPJ Digit Med. 2023;6(1):170.
12. Wang CS, FitzGerald JM, Schulzer M, Mak E, Ayas NT. Does this dyspneic patient in the emergency department have congestive heart failure? JAMA. 2005;294(15):1944–56.
13. Stein PD, Hull RD, Patel KC, Olson RE, Ghali WA, Brant R, et al. D-dimer for the exclusion of acute venous thrombosis and pulmonary embolism: a systematic review. Ann Intern Med. 2004;140(8):589–602.
14. Hicks SA, Strümke I, Thambawita V, Hammou M, Riegler MA, Halvorsen P, et al. On evaluation metrics for medical applications of artificial intelligence. Sci Rep. 2022;12(1):5979.
15. Hand D, Christen P. A note on using the F-measure for evaluating record linkage algorithms. Stat Comput. 2018;28:539–47.
16. Chicco D, Jurman G. The advantages of the Matthews correlation coefficient (MCC) over F1 score and accuracy in binary classification evaluation. BMC Genomics. 2020;21(1):6.
17. Cummings P. The relative merits of risk ratios and odds ratios. Arch Pediatr Adolesc Med. 2009;163(5):438–45.
18. Cook RJ, Sackett DL. The number needed to treat: a clinically useful measure of treatment effect. BMJ. 1995;310(6977):452–4.
19. Zermansky A. Number needed to harm should be measured for treatments. BMJ. 1998;317(7164):1014.
20. Sackett DL. The rational clinical examination. A primer on the precision and accuracy of the clinical examination. JAMA. 1992;267(19):2638–44.
21. Kent P, Hancock MJ. Interpretation of dichotomous outcomes: sensitivity, specificity, likelihood ratios, and pre-test and post-test probability. J Physiother. 2016;62(4):231–3.
22. Mandrekar JN. Receiver operating characteristic curve in diagnostic test assessment. J Thorac Oncol. 2010;5(9):1315–6.
23. Donaldson MS, Corrigan JM, Kohn LT. To err is human: building a safer health system. Washington, DC: The National Academies Press; 2000.
24. Jenniskens K, De Groot JA, Reitsma JB, Moons KG, Hooft L, Naaktgeboren CA. Overdiagnosis across medical disciplines: a scoping review. BMJ Open. 2017;7(12):e018448.
25. Falagas M, Vardakas K, Vergidis P. Under-diagnosis of common chronic diseases: prevalence and impact on human health. Int J Clin Pract. 2007;61(9):1569–79.
26. Institute of Medicine Committee on Quality of Health Care in A. 2 Improving the 21st-century health care system. Crossing the quality chasm: a new health system for the 21st century. Washington, DC: National Academies Press (US); 2001.
27. Yang D, Fineberg HV, Cosby K. Diagnostic excellence. JAMA. 2021;326(19):1905–6.
28. Berwick DM. Diagnostic excellence through the lens of patient-centeredness. JAMA. 2021;326(21):2127–8.

29. Singh H, Connor DM, Dhaliwal G. Five strategies for clinicians to advance diagnostic excellence. BMJ. 2022;376:e068044.
30. Neha D, Bui S, Morgan C, Hickey S, Paul CL. Interventions targeted at reducing diagnostic error: systematic review. BMJ Qual Saf. 2022;31(4):297–307.
31. Organization WH. Global patient safety report 2024. Geneva: World Health Organization; 2024.
32. Prevention CfDCa. Core elements of hospital diagnostic excellence (DxEx). 2025 [cited 2025 May 13]. Available from: https://www.cdc.gov/patient-safety/hcp/hospital-dx-excellence/index.html.
33. Morgan DJ, Singh H, Srinivasan A, Bradford A, McDonald LC, Kutty PK. CDC's core elements to promote diagnostic excellence. Diagnosis (Berl). 2024;12(2):197–200.

Historical Evolution of Diagnostic Techniques

2

Abstract

This chapter explores the historical evolution of diagnostic techniques, highlighting the dynamic interplay between technological innovation and clinical need. It provides an in-depth analysis of the transition from traditional methods like history taking and physical examination to modern advancements such as imaging and laboratory investigations. Additionally, it examines the transformative impact of artificial intelligence on diagnostics, tracing its development through periods of progress, challenges, and resurgence. By integrating traditional approaches with cutting-edge artificial intelligence-driven innovations, this chapter highlights the advancements shaping the future of precision medicine and healthcare delivery.

Keywords

Diagnostic techniques · Artificial intelligence · Medical imaging · Machine learning · Natural language processing · Transformer · Wearable devices · Precision medicine

2.1 Timeline of Historical Events in Diagnostic Methods and Artificial Intelligence

The journey of diagnostic techniques in medicine represents a dynamic interaction between technological innovation and clinical demand to improve patient care. This chapter highlights the progression of diagnostic methods, from foundational tools used long before the advent of artificial intelligence to the transformative impact of artificial intelligence on modern diagnostics. The timeline of representative events in diagnostic methods and artificial intelligence is summarized in Table 2.1.

T. Hirosawa, *Artificial Intelligence in Medical Diagnostics*,
https://doi.org/10.1007/978-981-95-4338-0_2

Table 2.1 Timeline of representative events in diagnostic methods and artificial intelligence (AI)

Timeline	Historical events in diagnostic methods	Artificial intelligence-related events
Before the 1800s	History taking is a major part of medical diagnostics	N/A
1816	Invention of the stethoscope by René Laennec, revolutionizing auscultation	N/A
1895	Discovery of X-rays by Wilhelm Conrad Röntgen, introducing internal imaging to medicine	N/A
1950	N/A	Alan Turing publishes "Computing Machinery and Intelligence," conceptualizing AI
1965	N/A	Development of ELIZA, one of the earliest natural language programs, demonstrating AI's conversational potential
1970s	Development of computed tomography (CT), providing detailed 3D anatomical insights	The Lighthill report (1973) and the first AI winter (1974–1980) due to computational limitations.
1980s	Introduction of magnetic resonance imaging (MRI), offering advanced imaging capabilities	Second AI winter (1987–1993) triggered by limitations of expert systems
1990s	Rise of handheld diagnostic tools, including portable ultrasounds	
2000s	Wearable diagnostic devices like echocardiography tools and smartwatches emerge	GPUs—and NVIDIA's Compute Unified Device Architecture (CUDA, 2007)—accelerated AI development
2010s	Widespread adoption of diagnostic imaging and	Resurgence of AI driven by neural networks and platforms like TensorFlow and PyTorch
2020s	wearable technologies	Release of powerful Generative Pretrained Transformer (GPT) models like ChatGPT, revolutionizing public access to AI (2022). Two Nobel Prizes highlighted AI's impact (e.g., in protein structure prediction) (2024)

2.2 Historical Evolution of Diagnostic Techniques Before Artificial Intelligence

Before the emergence of artificial intelligence, diagnostic techniques were grounded in the principles of history taking, physical examination, and advancements in imaging and laboratory investigations. These traditional approaches provided the groundwork for modern diagnostic practices, enabling healthcare professionals to systematically gather and interpret clinical information about patients' conditions. These traditional approaches, including history taking and physical examination, were rapidly becoming a lost art due to advancements in medical technologies [1–3]. However, a revisitation of these methods has occurred with the emergence of artificial intelligence, as detailed in Chap. 9.

2.2.1 History Taking

History taking is one of the oldest and most powerful diagnostic tools in clinical medicine [4]. Despite significant advancements in medical technologies, it remains fundamental to understand the patient's narrative [5]. Several landmark studies demonstrated that approximately 80% of diagnoses could be made based solely on a thorough medical history [6, 7]. Despite its importance, history taking is not without limitations. Its reliability can vary significantly, as it depends on the experience, communication skills, and clinical judgment of the healthcare professional. Moreover, patient factors such as recall bias, language barriers, and willingness to disclose information can further influence the quality of history obtained. By carefully gathering history, healthcare professionals formulate a post-history probability that guides subsequent diagnostic steps [8].

2.2.2 Stethoscope

Auscultation is an important component of the physical examination [9, 10]. The invention of the stethoscope by René Laennec in 1816 revolutionized the physical examination, particularly the practice of auscultation [11]. This iconic device enabled healthcare professionals to auscultate internal body sounds, such as cardiac sounds, pulmonary sounds, intestinal sounds, and vascular sounds. It provided valuable insights into a patient's condition. For example, the detection of murmurs or crackles could indicate cardiac valve abnormalities or pulmonary infections, respectively [9, 12]. Although the stethoscope has evolved over time, incorporating features like recording and amplification as digital stethoscopes [13], its core purpose remains unchanged [2].

2.2.3 X-ray Imaging

The discovery of X-rays by Wilhelm Conrad Röntgen in 1895 marked a milestone, enabling healthcare professionals to visualize internal structures no-invasively for the first time. This breakthrough laid the foundation for subsequent imaging technologies like computed tomography (CT) scans and allowed for the diagnosis of fractures and infections by revealing skeletal and soft tissue abnormalities. X-ray imaging quickly became a cornerstone of medical diagnostics and continues to be widely used today [14].

2.2.4 Laboratory Investigation

Laboratory investigations have been instrumental in augmenting diagnostic capabilities by providing quantitative and qualitative analyses of biological samples. Techniques such as blood tests, urinalysis, and microbiological cultures allow health care professionals to detect biochemical imbalances, infections, and organ dysfunctions [15]. For example, the development of serum hemoglobin testing revolutionized the diagnosis and management of anemia. For infectious diseases, microbiological techniques such as Gram staining and cultures remain essential to identify bacterial pathogens and guide antimicrobial therapy. With time, laboratory diagnostics have expanded to include advanced molecular techniques, such as polymerase chain reaction [16] and next-generation sequencing [17], which are pivotal in diagnosing infectious diseases and genetic conditions with high precision.

2.2.5 Computed Tomography and Magnetic Resonance Imaging

The advent of computed tomography in the 1970s and magnetic resonance imaging in the 1980s introduced three-dimensional imaging to medicine. Computer tomography scans utilize X-rays to produce detailed cross-sectional images, making them invaluable for diagnosing diseases such as trauma and tumors. Magnetic resonance imaging, on the other hand, uses powerful magnetic fields and radiofrequency waves to generate detailed images of soft tissues, making it ideal for detecting brain tumors, spinal cord injuries, and joint abnormalities. These modalities provided detailed anatomical and functional insights, facilitating the diagnosis of complex conditions [18, 19].

2.2.6 Handheld and Wearable Diagnostic Tools

Recent advancements in miniaturization and portability have led to the development of handheld ultrasound devices and wearable diagnostic tools. Handheld ultrasound devices, for example, enable real-time imaging at the bedside, allowing healthcare professionals to perform procedures like echocardiography and abdominal ultrasounds. These tools are particularly valuable at the point-of-care and in resource-limited or emergency settings [20, 21].

Wearable devices, such as smartwatches and fitness trackers, continuously monitor vital signs, including heart rate, blood oxygen saturation, and activity levels. These tools are increasingly being used to detect arrhythmias, track recovery in chronic conditions, and provide early warnings for conditions like sleep apnea or hypoxemia [22]. The integration of wearable technologies with mobile applications and cloud-based systems has enabled remote monitoring, empowering patients and enhancing chronic disease management [23].

To summarize, the historical evolution of diagnostic techniques before the advent of artificial intelligence illustrates humanity's ingenuity in addressing medical challenges through technology. These innovations laid a strong foundation for the transformative changes brought about by artificial intelligence, which are explored in the following sections.

2.3 Historical Evolution of Diagnostic Techniques with Artificial Intelligence

The integration of artificial intelligence into diagnostic techniques represents a transformative era in medical history. This paradigm shift has been driven by rapid advancements in computational power, the evolution of machine learning algorithms, and the advent of neural network techniques. Artificial intelligence has not only augmented traditional medical practices but also paved the way for a new era of precision medicine. This section traces the journey of artificial intelligence in medical diagnostics, from the conceptual beginnings to its modern applications.

2.3.1 Historical Evolution of Artificial Intelligence

Throughout history, technological innovations, such as the discovery of electricity, the harnessing of the transistor, the development of semiconductors, and the invention of the computer, have significantly altered human progress and reshaped societies [24]. These milestones not only revolutionized their respective domains but also catalyzed broader transformations in science, industry, and culture.

The comparison between artificial intelligence and pivotal historical innovations is not merely academic. It highlights artificial intelligence's potential to redefine industries, including healthcare. Like the industrial revolution, which mechanized production and changed the dynamics of labor, artificial intelligence has the capability to automate and optimize processes previously reliant on human expertise. This is particularly evident in medicine, where artificial intelligence has the potential to enable new diagnostic methodologies, predictive models, and personalized medicine. Artificial intelligence's impact may ultimately prove comparable to these innovations.

2.3.2 Foundation of Artificial Intelligence

The conceptual groundwork for artificial intelligence was laid in the mid-twentieth century, with Alan Turing being one of its most influential pioneers [25]. In 1950, Turing published his landmark paper, "Computing Machinery and Intelligence," which proposed the famous Turing Test, a method for determining whether a machine can exhibit intelligent behavior indistinguishable from that of a human. While Turing's ideas were primarily theoretical, they sparked a wave of interest in developing machines capable of performing tasks that required human-like intelligence. His work established a foundation for subsequent advancements in computer science and artificial intelligence.

In 1965, the development of ELIZA, one of the earliest natural language programs, demonstrated artificial intelligence's potential in mimicking human interaction. Created by Joseph Weizenbaum, ELIZA simulated a psychotherapist by engaging users in conversation [26]. Although ELIZA was not designed for medical diagnostics, its conversational ability revealed the possibilities of artificial intelligence in fields requiring human-like communication, paving the way for more sophisticated systems in healthcare.

The early enthusiasm for artificial intelligence was marked by optimism, with researchers envisioning machines capable of solving complex problems, learning from data, and even reasoning like humans. However, these expectations often outpaced the technological and computational capabilities of the time.

2.3.3 Artificial Intelligence Winter

Despite promising beginnings, artificial intelligence development faced challenges that led to several distinct periods of stagnation known as the artificial intelligence winters. In the context of artificial intelligence, the term "winter" refers to a prolonged phase of reduced public expectation, declining research support, and stagnation in industrial growth [27]. These winters resulted from a combination of unmet expectations, technical limitations, and economic constraints. The two main artificial intelligence winters occurred between 1974–1980 and 1987–1993 [28].

The first artificial intelligence winter arose from inflated expectations during the 1960s and early 1970s. Researchers promised breakthroughs in machine intelligence, but the available technology was not advanced enough to deliver on these promises. Early artificial intelligence systems relied heavily on rule-based programming, which required human developers to encode explicit instructions for every possible scenario. This approach proved inadequate for addressing the complexity and variability of real-world problems. Additionally, the computational power needed to support artificial intelligence research was limited, and datasets were often biased, incomplete, or insufficient for meaningful machine learning.

Government funding, which had fueled much of the early artificial intelligence research, began to dwindle as policymakers and stakeholders grew skeptical of the field's potential. Projects like the Lighthill Report in the UK criticized artificial intelligence research for its lack of real achievement, leading to decreased investment [29]. This downturn marked the first major setback for artificial intelligence development.

The second artificial intelligence winter occurred in the late 1980s and early 1990s, following another surge of optimism driven by advancements in expert systems. These systems attempted to encode human expertise into computer programs, offering decision support in areas such as diagnostics, engineering, and finance. However, the limitations of expert systems soon became apparent. They were expensive to build and maintain, and their performance was restricted to narrowly defined domains.

A notable example of failure during this period was Japan's Fifth Generation Computer Systems Project [30]. Launched in the early 1980s with ambitious goals of creating artificial intelligence-driven machines capable of reasoning and learning, the project ultimately fell short of its objectives. The lack of substantial progress led to widespread disillusionment, prompting governments and private institutions to withdraw funding for artificial intelligence initiatives.

2.3.4 Why Did Artificial Intelligence Fail During These Periods?

Several key factors contributed to the setbacks experienced during the artificial intelligence winters. One major bottleneck was inadequate data. Early artificial intelligence systems lacked access to large, high-quality datasets, making it difficult for machines to generalize or learn effectively. For instance, an illustrative example of biased training data comes from early computer vision experiments where an artificial intelligence model was trained to identify vehicles in images. Instead of learning the specific features of vehicles, the model differentiated between sunny and cloudy days [31]. Technological constraints also played a role [32]; limited computational power, especially in the pre-Graphics Processing Units (GPUs) era, hindered the development of complex algorithms and neural networks. Additionally, human bias influenced artificial intelligence development, as models were often constrained by the narrow and strict rule-based instructions encoded by their developers. Systems like MYCIN, designed for infectious diseases consultation, failed to perform well in diverse real-world scenarios [33, 34], as detailed in Chap. 3.

Despite these challenges, the artificial intelligence winters were not periods of complete stagnation. Instead, they provided an opportunity for researchers to reflect on the limitations of early approaches and develop the theoretical and practical tools needed for artificial intelligence's eventual resurgence [35].

2.3.5 Spring in Artificial Intelligence

Recent decades have marked a springtime for artificial intelligence, characterized by a resurgence of interest, investment, and innovation in the field. This renewed momentum has been driven by advancements in computational power, the development of sophisticated algorithms, and the widespread availability of accessible development platforms [27]. Together, these factors have propelled artificial intelligence from the theoretical and experimental stages into real-world applications across diverse industries, including healthcare.

2.4 Representative Milestone in Generative Artificial Intelligence

2.4.1 Machine Learning and Deep Learning

Machine learning introduced a paradigm shift by enabling systems to learn from data rather than relying solely on predefined rules. Within machine learning, deep learning represents a subset that uses artificial neural networks with multiple layers to model complex patterns. This development brought significant advancements in image recognition, natural language processing, and predictive analytics. These terms in artificial intelligence context are discussed in Chap. 4. In healthcare, machine learning and deep learning have transformed the field by enabling technologies such as diagnostic imaging systems that detect anomalies in X-rays or magnetic resonance imaging and predictive models that forecast patient outcomes based on comprehensive datasets.

2.4.2 Graphics Processing Units, Natural Language Processing, and Large Language Models

One of the most transformative advancements in this artificial intelligence renaissance has been the development of GPUs. Originally designed for rendering high-quality graphics in gaming and visual simulations, GPUs have proven to be ideal for the parallel processing required in training complex neural networks. In 2007, NVIDIA released Compute Unified Device Architecture, a general-purpose GPU programming framework. These technological advancements made it feasible to train large language models (LLMs), which underpin many modern artificial intelligence applications [36]. For instance, certain neural networks that once required weeks of computation on traditional Central Processing Units (CPUs) can currently be trained within hours using GPUs.

The rise in user-friendly development platforms like TensorFlow and PyTorch has further accelerated this progress. TensorFlow is renowned for its scalability and comprehensive ecosystem, making it ideal for both beginners and advanced users. On the other hand, PyTorch is favored for its dynamic computation graph, which offers greater flexibility and ease of debugging, particularly during research and experimentation. Together, these platforms have lowered barriers to entry and expanded the accessibility of artificial intelligence development across industries. These tools simplify the process of building, training, and deploying artificial intelligence models, making advanced artificial intelligence techniques accessible even to non-expert developers. TensorFlow, developed by the Google Brain team, and PyTorch, developed by Meta (formerly Facebook) AI Research, have become indispensable in artificial intelligence research and industry applications [37, 38]. They have offered pre-built libraries, intuitive interfaces, and community support. The details of TensorFlow and PyTorch were explained in Chap. 4.

2.4.3 Transformer Models and Generative Pretrained Transformers

Additionally, accessible development platforms, such as cloud-based services, have further expanded the reach of artificial intelligence by enabling developers to utilize scalable resources without the need for expensive on-premises infrastructure. Chat-style interfaces integrated into these platforms have also improved usability, allowing both technical and non-technical users to interact with artificial intelligence models and streamline their workflows [39].

The introduction of transformer models in 2017 marked a breakthrough in handling sequential data, revolutionizing natural language processing. The Generative Pretrained Transformer (GPT) architecture, developed by OpenAI, capitalized on this innovation. ChatGPT was released in November 2022, quickly becoming a popular generative AI platform. The GPT-3 series was later deprecated as newer versions were released, further solidifying OpenAI's position in AI advancements. GPT models learn language representations from vast amounts of text data, enabling them to generate coherent and contextually accurate text. Subsequent iterations, such as GPT-4 and its multimodal variants, introduced stronger reasoning and the ability to process images and audio, making these models widely useful tools [40, 41]. For healthcare professionals, applications range from summarizing medical literature and generating patient reports to facilitating patient-provider communication through chatbot interfaces. The potential for unspecialized generative AI for medical diagnostics is discussed in Chap. 5. Some researchers have referred to recent artificial intelligence innovation as the Fourth Industrial Revolution and have identified the impact of these innovations on how we work and live [42, 43].

A key figure in the artificial intelligence renaissance is Professor Geoffrey Hinton, often referred to as the "Godfather of Artificial Intelligence." His groundbreaking work on neural networks, including backpropagation and deep learning, has laid the foundation for modern artificial intelligence systems [44]. Hinton's contributions have not only advanced the theoretical understanding of machine learning but also paved the way for practical applications in fields such as computer vision, natural language processing, and digital health. In 2024, two Nobel Prizes recognized AI-related contributions in physics and chemistry. Mainstream media—including pieces like "A Shift in the World of Science"—highlighted the technology's broad impact on science and society [45].

In summary, these historical developments illustrate the profound evolution of diagnostic techniques, from traditional tools to artificial intelligence-driven innovations. The spring of artificial intelligence has brought about breakthroughs that have revolutionized diagnostics, enhancing accuracy, efficiency, and accessibility. By integrating artificial intelligence into healthcare, medical diagnostics are entering a new era of precision medicine, where treatments and interventions are tailored to individual patients. These systems excel at analyzing complex datasets, integrating radiological images with patient history and laboratory results to offer a holistic diagnostic view. Such applications extend to generating personalized treatment plans by synthesizing genetic, clinical, and behavioral data, thus enhancing decision-making capabilities.

References

1. Chizner MA. Cardiac auscultation: rediscovering the lost art. Curr Probl Cardiol. 2008;33(7):326–408.
2. Bank I, Vliegen HW, Bruschke AV. The 200th anniversary of the stethoscope: can this low-tech device survive in the high-tech 21st century? Eur Heart J. 2016;37(47):3536–43.

3. Schechter GP, Blank LL, Godwin HA, LaCombe MA, Novack DH, Rosse WF. Refocusing on history-taking skills during Internal Medicine Training. Am J Med. 1996;101(2):210–6.
4. Stoeckle JD, Billings JA. A history of history-taking: the medical interview. J Gen Intern Med. 1987;2(2):119–27.
5. Lichstein PR. The medical interview. In: Walker HKHW, Hurst JW, editors. Clinical methods: the history, physical, and laboratory examinations. 3rd ed. Boston: Butterworths; 1990.
6. Hampton JR, Harrison MJ, Mitchell JR, Prichard JS, Seymour C. Relative contributions of history-taking, physical examination, and laboratory investigation to diagnosis and management of medical outpatients. Br Med J. 1975;2(5969):486–9.
7. Peterson MC, Holbrook JH, Von Hales D, Smith NL, Staker LV. Contributions of the history, physical examination, and laboratory investigation in making medical diagnoses. West J Med. 1992;156(2):163–5.
8. Summerton N. The medical history as a diagnostic technology. Br J Gen Pract. 2008;58(549):273–6.
9. Bohadana A, Izbicki G, Kraman SS. Fundamentals of lung auscultation. N Engl J Med. 2014;370(8):744–51.
10. Pelech AN. The physiology of cardiac auscultation. Pediatr Clin N Am. 2004;51(6):1515–35.
11. Morris JS. Laennec's stethoscope—the Welsh connection. J R Soc Med. 2004;97(3):137–41.
12. Phua K, Chen J, Dat TH, Shue L. Heart sound as a biometric. Pattern Recogn. 2008;41(3):906–19.
13. Kalinauskienė E, Razvadauskas H, Morse DJ, Maxey GE, Naudžiūnas A. A comparison of electronic and traditional stethoscopes in the heart auscultation of obese patients. Medicina (Kaunas). 2019;55(4):94.
14. Panchbhai AS. Wilhelm Conrad Röntgen and the discovery of X-rays: revisited after centennial. J Indian Acad Oral Med Radiol. 2015;27(1):90–5.
15. Lippi G. The origin of some laboratory medicine milestones. J Lab Precis Med. 2019;4:14.
16. Kubista M, Andrade JM, Bengtsson M, Forootan A, Jonák J, Lind K, et al. The real-time polymerase chain reaction. Mol Aspects Med. 2006;27(2):95–125.
17. Hu T, Chitnis N, Monos D, Dinh A. Next-generation sequencing technologies: an overview. Hum Immunol. 2021;82(11):801–11.
18. Wesolowski JR, Lev MH. CT: history, technology, and clinical aspects. Semin Ultrasound CT MRI. 2005;26(6):376–9.
19. Runge VM. Current technological advances in magnetic resonance with critical impact for clinical diagnosis and therapy. Investig Radiol. 2013;48(12):869–77.
20. Andersen CA, Holden S, Vela J, Rathleff MS, Jensen MB. Point-of-care ultrasound in general practice: a systematic review. Ann Fam Med. 2019;17(1):61–9.
21. Popat A, Harikrishnan S, Seby N, Sen U, Patel SK, Mittal L, et al. Utilization of point-of-care ultrasound as an imaging modality in the emergency department: a systematic review and meta-analysis. Cureus. 2024;16(1):e52371.
22. Wang Y-C, Xu X, Hajra A, Apple S, Kharawala A, Duarte G, et al. Current advancement in diagnosing atrial fibrillation by utilizing wearable devices and artificial intelligence: a review study. Diagnostics. 2022;12(3):689.
23. Chakraborty A, Islam M, Shahriyar F, Islam S, Zaman HU, Hasan M. Smart home system: a comprehensive review. J Electr Comput Eng. 2023;2023(1):7616683.
24. Miller C. Chip war: the fight for the world's most critical technology. New York City: Simon and Schuster; 2022.
25. Turing AM. Computing machinery and intelligence. Mind. 1950;59:433–60.
26. Weizenbaum J. ELIZA—a computer program for the study of natural language communication between man and machine. Commun ACM. 1966;9(1):36–45.
27. Delipetrev B, Tsinaraki C, Kostic U. Historical evolution of artificial intelligence. Luxembourg: Publications Office of the European Union; 2020.
28. Aliferis C, Simon G. Lessons learned from historical failures, limitations and successes of AI/ML in healthcare and the health sciences. Enduring problems, and the role of best practices.

In: Simon GJ, Aliferis C, editors. Artificial intelligence and machine learning in health care and medical sciences: best practices and pitfalls. Cham: Springer International Publishing; 2024. p. 543–606.

29. Lighthill J. Artificial intelligence: a general survey. In: Science Research Council, artificial intelligence: a paper symposium. London: SRC; 1973. p. 21.
30. Garvey CS. "AI for social good" and the first AI arms race lessons from Japan's fifth generation computer systems (FGCS) project. The Japanese Society for Artificial Intelligence. 2020;JSAI2020:2O1ES501-2O1ES.
31. Dreyfus HL, Dreyfus SE. What artificial experts can and cannot do. AI Soc. 1992;6(1):18–26.
32. Mead C, Conway L. Introduction to VLSI systems. Reading: Addison-Wesley; 1980.
33. Yu VL, Fagan LM, Wraith SM, Clancey WJ, Scott AC, Hannigan J, et al. Antimicrobial selection by a computer: a blinded evaluation by infectious diseases experts. JAMA. 1979;242(12):1279–82.
34. Davis R. Consultation, knowledge acquisition, and instruction: a case study. In: Chapter 3 in Szolovits P, editor. Artificial intelligence in medicine. Colorado: Westview Press; 1982. p. 57–78.
35. Adamopoulou E, Moussiades L. Chatbots: history, technology, and applications. Mach Learn Appl. 2020;2:100006.
36. Pandey M, Fernandez M, Gentile F, Isayev O, Tropsha A, Stern AC, et al. The transformational role of GPU computing and deep learning in drug discovery. Nat Mach Intell. 2022;4(3):211–21.
37. Akkisetty PK. An overview of AI platforms, frameworks, libraries, and processors. In: Rahmani AM, Raj CP, Nagasubramanian G, Ranganath S, Colby R, editors. Model optimization methods for efficient and edge AI: federated learning architectures, frameworks and applications. Hoboken: Wiley; 2024. p. 43–55.
38. Paszke A. Pytorch: an imperative style, high-performance deep learning library. arXiv preprint arXiv:191201703. 2019.
39. Wang YC, Xue J, Wei C, Kuo CCJ. An overview on generative AI at scale with edge–cloud computing. IEEE Open J Commun Soc. 2023;4:2952–71.
40. OpenAI. OpenAI o1 System Card. arXiv preprint. 2024;arXiv:2412:16720.
41. OpenAI. OpenAI o3-mini System Card 2025 [updated January 31]. Available from: https://cdn.openai.com/o3-mini-system-card.pdf.
42. Chakraborty U, Banerjee A, Saha JK, Sarkar N, Chakraborty C. Artificial intelligence and the fourth industrial revolution. Boca Raton, FL: CRC Press; 2022.
43. Chaka C. Fourth industrial revolution—a review of applications, prospects, and challenges for artificial intelligence, robotics and blockchain in higher education. Res Pract Technol Enhanc Learn. 2023;18:002.
44. Krizhevsky A, Sutskever I, Hinton GE. Imagenet classification with deep convolutional neural networks. Adv Neural Inf Process Syst. 2012;25. https://doi.org/10.1145/3065386.
45. Li B, Gilbert S. Artificial Intelligence awarded two Nobel Prizes for innovations that will shape the future of medicine. npj Digit Med. 2024;7(1):336.

Overview of Diagnostic Clinical Decision Support Systems

3

Abstract

This chapter provides a comprehensive exploration of Clinical Decision Support Systems (CDSSs), with a particular emphasis on diagnostic CDSS. The primary aim is to delineate the various classifications and functionalities of CDSSs while highlighting their pivotal role in modern health care. By exploring the methodologies underlying diagnostic CDSS—knowledge-based and non-knowledge-based—this chapter emphasizes their contributions to clinical workflows, their strengths and limitations, and their potential to improve diagnostic accuracy, efficiency, and patient outcomes. Additionally, specialized diagnostic CDSS applications in laboratory, imaging, and pathology contexts are explored, illustrating how these systems integrate advanced technologies to transform the diagnostic landscape.

Keywords

Clinical decision support systems · Knowledge-based systems · Non-knowledge based systems · Diagnostic accuracy · Symptom checkers · Differential diagnosis generators

3.1 Classification of Clinical Decision Support Systems

Clinical Decision Support Systems (CDSSs) are computer-based tools designed to aid health-care professionals in making clinical decisions. CDSSs are effective at improving health-care process measures across diverse settings [1]. CDSSs can be categorized based on two primary dimensions: their primary function, such as diagnostic support versus other applications, and their reliance on predefined knowledge versus data-driven models [2]. This chapter focuses specifically on diagnostic CDSSs, a subset of CDSSs that prioritize supporting health-care professionals in

T. Hirosawa, *Artificial Intelligence in Medical Diagnostics*,
https://doi.org/10.1007/978-981-95-4338-0_3

the diagnostic process. It further explores how these systems differ in their underlying methodologies: knowledge-based and non-knowledge-based systems.

3.2 Diagnostic Clinical Decision Support Systems in Clinical Decision Support Systems

While CDSS encompasses a broad range of functionalities, diagnostic CDSS specifically focuses on assisting health-care professionals in formulating diagnoses. Other types of CDSS serve equally vital functions in health-care delivery, extending their impact across therapeutic, preventative, and administrative domains. This section focuses on diagnostic CDSSs.

3.2.1 Diagnostic Clinical Decision Support Systems

Diagnostic support, in general, refers to any process or tool that facilitates the identification of a patient's condition or illness. This can range from simple algorithms to complex machine learning methods that analyze patient data to suggest differential diagnosis.

3.2.2 Specialized Diagnostic Clinical Decision Support Systems

Specialized diagnostic CDSS represents advanced technological tools designed to enhance the diagnostic process across various clinical domains. These systems facilitate the extraction, visualization, and interpretation of laboratory test results, medical images, and pathological data. By integrating seamlessly into clinical workflows, diagnostic CDSSs provide actionable insights, improve diagnostic accuracy, and reduce the workload of health-care professionals.

In the context of clinical reasoning and differential diagnosis, specialized diagnostic CDSSs serve a pivotal function by integrating diverse clinical data and applying evidence-based algorithms. These systems assist health-care professionals in systematically considering a wide spectrum of potential diagnoses, including rare diseases or atypical presentations. By correlating patient symptoms with laboratory values, imaging results, and pathological features, CDSSs facilitate comprehensive diagnostic assessments. This structured analytical approach reduces the cognitive burden on health-care professionals, prioritizes diagnostic possibilities, recommends targeted investigations, and supports the development of personalized clinical strategies [3].

In laboratory medicine, diagnostic CDSS plays a potential role in analyzing and interpreting laboratory results. For instance, they can automatically detect abnormal blood test values and correlate these findings with potential underlying conditions by referencing established clinical guidelines or utilizing predictive models. Beyond simple identification of abnormalities, these systems can integrate multiple laboratory parameters to deliver a comprehensive interpretation that supports the formulation of differential diagnoses and the next step [4].

In the fields of medical imaging, diagnostic CDSS assists health-care professionals, particularly radiologists. These systems can highlight suspicious areas on imaging modalities such as X-rays, computed tomography scans, or magnetic resonance imaging. By suggesting potential interpretations based on image features, they assist health-care professionals in identifying and characterizing abnormalities. Furthermore, advanced systems can automatically measure or quantify specific features—such as lesion size, tissue density, or organ volume—improving both diagnostic accuracy and efficiency. This capability is beneficial in complex or time-sensitive cases where timely decision-making is essential to effective patient care [5].

In pathology, diagnostic CDSS offers transformative potential through the analysis of digitized tissue samples. These systems can identify patterns and features indicative of specific diseases, such as the presence of malignant cells or inflammatory processes. Additionally, they assist pathologists in grading and staging tumors, providing objective metrics that enhance reproducibility and consistency in diagnostic evaluations [6].

Specialized diagnostic CDSSs streamline the diagnostic process by automating repetitive tasks, reducing human error, and enabling health care professionals to focus on higher-level clinical decision-making. By enhancing diagnostic accuracy and efficiency, these systems contribute significantly to improving the outcome of patient care and supporting the broader goals of precision medicine.

3.3 Knowledge-Based Clinical Decision Support Systems and Non-knowledge-Based Clinical Decision Support Systems

This section explores the two broad categories of CDSS's underlying methodologies: knowledge-based CDSS and non-knowledge-based CDSS. While some researchers classified rule-based CDSS and machine learning-based CDSS [7], this book adopts the classification of knowledge-based CDSS and non-knowledge-based CDSS. The comparison is shown in Table 3.1.

3.3.1 Knowledge-Based Clinical Decision Support Systems

Knowledge-based CDSS relies on predefined rules and structured medical knowledge. These systems encode clinical guidelines, expert opinions, and established protocols into their frameworks. By following logical rules and clinical algorithms, they provide consistent and explainable recommendations. This approach ensures that the recommendations are transparent and based on well-understood medical knowledge. Common examples include MYCIN, symptom checkers, and traditional differential-diagnosis generators, which assist both the public and health-care professionals.

Table 3.1 Comparison of knowledge-based clinical decision support system (CDSS) and non-knowledge-based CDSS

Aspect	Knowledge-based CDSS	Non-knowledge-based CDSS
Type	Based on fixed rules and expert medical knowledge	Data-driven models that rely on artificial intelligence (AI), machine learning, and statistical pattern recognition
Examples	MYCIN, Symptom Checkers, Traditional Differential-Diagnosis Generators such as DXplain®	Watson, Isabel Pro, Med Gemini
Purpose	Assist with triage and diagnostic reasoning	Support medical diagnostics through pattern recognition
Inputs	Patient-reported symptoms for symptom checkers; detailed clinical data for differential-diagnosis generators	Clinical manifestations
Outputs	List of potential conditions with guidance or differential diagnoses with reasoning	Differential diagnoses or task-specific recommendations
Strengths	Accessible to the public for symptom checkers, comprehensive analysis for differential-diagnosis generators	Potentially higher accuracy and adaptability due to AI; generative AI advancements
Weaknesses	Inadequate accuracy, reliance on structured inputs, often time-consuming, and difficult integration with clinical workflows	Lack of explainability, negative perceptions among professionals, inadequate accuracy in some cases, and reliance on manual data entry without integration into health systems

3.3.2 Knowledge-Based Clinical Decision Support Systems: MYCIN

MYCIN is one of the earliest knowledge-based CDSSs developed in the 1970s at Stanford University. It was specifically designed to assist in the diagnosis and treatment of infectious diseases [8–10]. The system used a rule-based approach, incorporating approximately 600 rules derived from expert knowledge in infectious diseases [11]. These rules were encoded into a knowledge base, and MYCIN employed an inference engine to analyze clinical data and generate diagnostic and therapeutic recommendations.

One of MYCIN's most notable features was its ability to explain its reasoning process. When providing a recommendation, the system could detail the rules it applied and the data it analyzed to reach a conclusion. This level of transparency was groundbreaking for its time, as it allowed health-care professionals to understand and potentially trust the system's recommendations. MYCIN's recommendations included identifying the most likely pathogens causing an infection and suggesting appropriate antibiotic treatments, taking into account patient-specific factors such as allergies [12].

Despite its innovative approach, MYCIN faced significant limitations that hindered its adoption in real clinical settings. One major challenge was the system's narrow focus on infectious diseases, which limited its applicability in broader medical contexts. Furthermore, MYCIN required users to input data manually, which was both time-consuming and prone to errors. Inconsistent data quality and the lack of integration with electronic health record systems further reduced its practical utility. Another significant barrier was resistance from health-care professionals, many of whom were hesitant to rely on a computer system for decision-making. This resistance, combined with the practical challenges of manual data entry, meant that MYCIN was never actually used in routine clinical practice, serving instead as a foundational research project.

Studies evaluating MYCIN's performance showed that its accuracy was comparable to that of infectious disease experts [13, 14]. However, its rigid rule-based structure also posed challenges. The system lacked the flexibility to adapt to new medical knowledge or to handle cases that fell outside its predefined knowledge base. Over time, this rigidity became a critical drawback as medical knowledge expanded and diversified.

MYCIN's legacy lies in its pioneering role in demonstrating the potential of computer-based decision support in medicine. Lessons learned from MYCIN's successes and shortcomings have informed the evolution of more sophisticated and adaptable CDSS, including those that integrate machine learning and advanced data analytics. In retrospect, MYCIN remains a landmark in the history of medical informatics, illustrating the promise and challenges of applying artificial intelligence in health care.

3.3.3 Knowledge-Based Clinical Decision Support Systems: Symptom Checkers

Symptom checkers are tools designed for public users to provide initial guidance regarding the urgency of seeking medical attention. These systems use patient-reported symptoms entered through guided interview formats and process them using rule-based approaches, decision trees, or Bayesian networks. The core function of a symptom checker is to map the symptoms to potential conditions, generating a list of possibilities accompanied by recommendations for next steps. These might include advice for self-care, recommendations to consult a health-care professional, or indicators of an emergency requiring immediate attention [15]. Figure 3.1 illustrates a sample interface of a symptom checker.

The primary strength of symptom checkers lies in their accessibility and ability to empower patients. They provide a first layer of guidance, allowing users to understand their symptoms and consider possible conditions before visiting a health-care professional. This can be particularly helpful in alleviating users' anxiety and directing patients to appropriate care pathways. However, symptom checkers are also not without limitations [16, 17]. Their accuracy can be inadequate due to their reliance on self-reported symptoms, which are often subjective or incomplete. Additionally, symptom checkers tend to focus on common conditions and may fail to reflect the complexity and variability of real-world clinical cases. Further

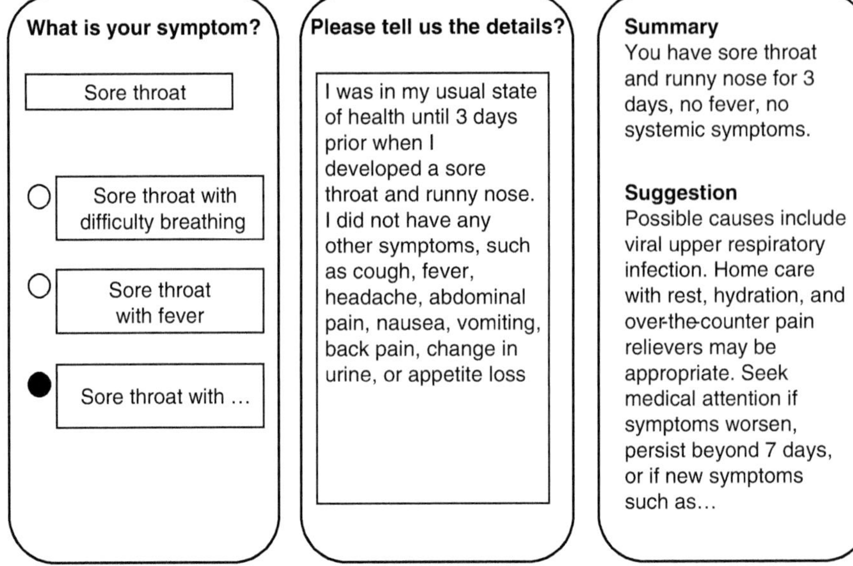

Fig. 3.1 Example interface of a symptom checker displayed across three smartphone-like screens

limitations arise from their reliance on fixed rules, which may lag current medical knowledge and require frequent updates to remain relevant.

3.3.4 Knowledge-Based Clinical Decision Support Systems: Traditional Differential-Diagnosis Generator

Traditional differential-diagnosis generators such as DXplain® are designed to assist health-care professionals by supporting their clinical reasoning process. These systems rely on detailed and specific inputs, including patient demographics, medical history, physical exam findings, and investigation results, to generate a prioritized list of potential diagnoses. Unlike symptom checkers, differential-diagnosis generators offer a more detailed analysis. They often incorporate evidence-based reasoning and provide specific explanations [18]. Figure 3.2 illustrates a sample interface of a traditional differential-diagnosis generator. The system displays an input panel where health-care professionals can enter patient details and clinical findings and an output section that presents a ranked list of possible diagnoses.

Systems like DXplain® are widely recognized in this category. It was developed by the University of Massachusetts in 1986. It exemplifies these systems as a rule-based reference tool that outputs differential diagnoses based on clinical manifestations provided by health-care professionals [19]. DXplain® uses advanced computational techniques to analyze symptoms and propose a list of differential diagnoses. Its utility has been supported by scientific evidence; for instance, a randomized controlled trial demonstrated significantly high diagnostic accuracy when

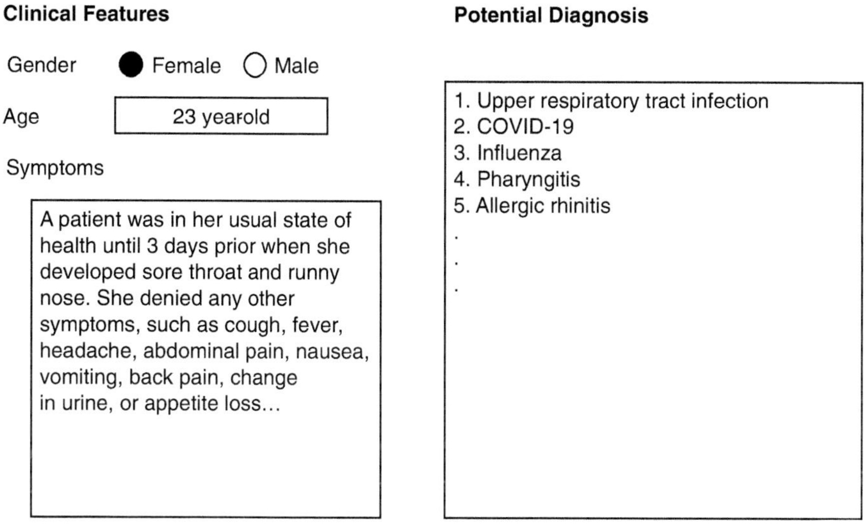

Clinical Features

Gender ● Female ○ Male

Age 23 yearold

Symptoms

A patient was in her usual state of health until 3 days prior when she developed sore throat and runny nose. She denied any other symptoms, such as cough, fever, headache, abdominal pain, nausea, vomiting, back pain, change in urine, or appetite loss...

Potential Diagnosis

1. Upper respiratory tract infection
2. COVID-19
3. Influenza
4. Pharyngitis
5. Allergic rhinitis

.
.
.

Fig. 3.2 Example interface of a traditional differential-diagnosis generator

used by health-care professionals during validated diagnosis tests [20]. Moreover, an additional study highlighted its ability to improve diagnostic quality while reducing costs in teaching hospitals [21]. These findings highlight the system's potential as an invaluable tool for clinical reasoning, especially in settings where accurate and efficient diagnostic processes are critical.

The primary strength of differential-diagnosis generators lies in their ability to provide comprehensive and explainable reasoning, particularly in complex cases where clinical decision-making can be challenging. By structuring the diagnostic process and systematically evaluating patient data, these systems encourage a thorough approach to diagnosis. They also help health-care professionals consider a broader range of possibilities, reducing the likelihood of missed or delayed diagnoses.

However, these systems also face limitations. A major challenge is their reliance on structured and high-quality input data; the completeness and accuracy of the data provided directly impact the system's performance. In real clinical settings, incomplete or inconsistent data may reduce their reliability. Additionally, integration with electronic health record (EHR) systems and other health-care technologies remains limited, which can create inefficiencies and hinder seamless use within clinical workflows. Generating differential diagnoses may also be time-consuming, which is a critical drawback in high-pressure, time-sensitive environments such as emergency departments, where rapid decision-making is essential.

In conclusion, knowledge-based CDSSs, including MYCIN, symptom checkers, and traditional differential-diagnosis generators, provide valuable support in both public and health-care professional contexts. Their effectiveness depends on the quality of data, the complexity of the cases, and their adaptability to evolving medical knowledge and technological integration. Additionally, they laid the groundwork for subsequent developments in CDSS by highlighting both the possibilities and limitations of knowledge-based systems [22].

3.3.5 Non-knowledge-Based Clinical Decision Support Systems

Non-knowledge-based CDSSs leverage artificial intelligence, machine learning, and statistical pattern recognition, rather than relying on predefined rules or expert medical knowledge. These systems aim to identify patterns in data and generate diagnostic recommendations and care plans based on the insights derived from computational models. Several examples of such systems include established IBM's Watson and Isabel Pro, as well as emerging generative artificial intelligence models like Med Gemini, which have been developed to assist health-care professionals.

3.3.6 Non-knowledge-Based Clinical Decision Support Systems: Watson

Watson, developed by IBM, represents one of the pioneering efforts in integrating artificial intelligence into medical diagnostics and clinical decision support. Leveraging its sophisticated natural language processing and machine learning capabilities, Watson was designed to process vast quantities of unstructured and structured medical data. The system aims to assist health-care professionals by synthesizing information from diverse medical literature, clinical guidelines, and patient-specific data to generate diagnostic insights and recommend evidence-based treatment options [23].

Watson for Oncology, developed in collaboration with leading cancer institutes, exemplifies the system's specialized applications. It assists oncologists by analyzing patient medical records alongside cancer treatment guidelines and literature. The system suggests treatment options ranked by efficacy and relevance, with accompanying evidence to support its recommendations. A systematic review demonstrated the overall concordance rate of 82% between the multidisciplinary team and Watson for Oncology [24]. Other studies supported by IBM claim concordance rates as high as 96% [25]. By highlighting suspicious regions and correlating findings with clinical data, Watson aids radiologists in diagnosing conditions like cancer, cardiovascular diseases, and neurological disorders. Its ability to process imaging data alongside clinical context enhances diagnostic accuracy and efficiency. In the context of rare disease diagnosis, Watson addresses challenges due to its complexity and low prevalence by analyzing vast datasets and identifying correlations that may elude health-care professionals. By generating differential diagnoses and suggesting additional tests, Watson facilitates earlier and more accurate identification of rare conditions.

Although there were several successful collaborations between hospitals and Watson, some collaborations resulted in failures [26]. Watson represents a groundbreaking innovation in the realm of non-knowledge-based clinical decision support systems. By harnessing the power of artificial intelligence, it has the potential to revolutionize medical diagnostics and decision-making. However, addressing its current challenges is critical to realizing its full potential and ensuring its adoption as a trusted tool in health care [27].

3.3.7 Non-knowledge-Based Clinical Decision Support Systems: Isabel Pro

Isabel Pro is another notable non-knowledge-based clinical decision support system designed to aid in diagnostic accuracy and efficiency. Developed by Isabel Healthcare, this system leverages machine learning algorithms to generate differential diagnoses based on the input of symptoms, patient demographics, and clinical findings. Isabel Pro's intuitive interface allows health-care professionals to input clinical data and receive a list of potential diagnoses ranked by relevance and likelihood [28].

One of the key features of Isabel Pro is its ability to incorporate a vast repository of medical knowledge, including rare diseases, which often pose significant diagnostic challenges. This capability makes Isabel Pro particularly valuable in settings where health-care professionals may encounter a broad spectrum of conditions, such as emergency departments or rural health-care facilities. Additionally, Isabel Pro integrates seamlessly with electronic health record systems by several vendors [28]. By streamlining data entry and automating parts of the diagnostic process, the system aims to reduce the cognitive burden on health-care professionals and improve diagnostic workflow efficiency.

An empirical study suggested that Isabel Pro produced 87% correct diagnoses for complex case series [29]. Another study documented the improvement (7–8%) in diagnostic accuracy of health-care professionals when using Isabel Pro [30]. The system has been credited with improving diagnostic accuracy in scenarios involving atypical presentations or rare conditions.

In terms of accessibility, Isabel Pro is often highlighted for its affordability and scalability, making it a viable option for smaller practices and under-resourced health-care facilities. The system's user-friendly design and compatibility with mobile devices further enhance its usability, allowing health-care professionals to access diagnostic support at the point of care.

However, it also shares common limitations with other non-knowledge-based systems, including a reliance on high-quality input data and the need for continuous updates to its algorithm to reflect advancements in medical knowledge. Additionally, like other artificial intelligence-driven systems, it faces issues related to transparency, as its underlying algorithms are not always fully disclosed to users. This lack of explainability may hinder health-care professional trust and adoption in certain settings.

Isabel Pro represents a promising tool in the landscape of non-knowledge-based clinical decision support systems. By combining advanced machine learning algorithms with a user-centric design, it has the potential to enhance diagnostic accuracy and efficiency across diverse clinical settings. Addressing challenges related to transparency, data integration, and algorithm updates will be critical to its continued success and broader adoption in the health-care sector.

3.3.8 Non-knowledge-Based Clinical Decision Support Systems: Med Gemini

Med Gemini, developed by Google AI, represents an advanced application of generative artificial intelligence in the field of clinical decision support. The system is trained on extensive medical resources and operates as part of the broader Gemini platform. A preliminary, non-peer-reviewed study has reported better accuracy in performing medical tasks compared to other non-specialized generative artificial intelligence systems [31]. This suggests that Med Gemini holds potential in revolutionizing clinical diagnostics and decision-making. However, access to this system remains limited to selected researchers, which restricts its validation and broader application in real clinical settings.

Despite the promising advancements in non-knowledge-based CDSS, their impact on clinical diagnosis has been less pronounced compared to other domains of medicine. Several challenges contribute to this limited influence. Their lack of explainability can make it difficult for health-care professionals to understand or trust their recommendations, a phenomenon often referred to as the "black box" problem [32]. Another significant issue is the negative perception among health-care professionals, often stemming from biases and lack of trust in artificial intelligence-driven systems. Additionally, these systems frequently suffer from inadequate accuracy, particularly in complex or ambiguous cases. Another major barrier is poor integration with existing health-care systems. Most non-knowledge-based CDSS requires manual data entry, which is time-consuming and disrupts clinical workflow efficiency, further discouraging adoption [33].

In conclusion, non-knowledge-based CDSSs, such as Watson, Isabel Pro, and Med Gemini, offer substantial potential to enhance medical diagnostics by leveraging artificial intelligence and pattern recognition capabilities. However, addressing the challenges of accuracy, system integration, and health-care professionals' perceptions is key for their broader acceptance and effective implementation in clinical practice. These systems remain in the developmental phase and are not yet fully mature for routine clinical deployment. Future research, cross-disciplinary collaboration, and iterative refinement will be essential to address these limitations and successfully integrate these powerful tools into the complex ecosystem of clinical practice.

References

1. Bright TJ, Wong A, Dhurjati R, Bristow E, Bastian L, Coeytaux RR, et al. Effect of clinical decision-support systems: a systematic review. Ann Intern Med. 2012;157(1):29–43.
2. Sutton RT, Pincock D, Baumgart DC, Sadowski DC, Fedorak RN, Kroeker KI. An overview of clinical decision support systems: benefits, risks, and strategies for success. NPJ Digit Med. 2020;3(1):17.

3. van Baalen S, Boon M, Verhoef P. From clinical decision support to clinical reasoning support systems. J Eval Clin Pract. 2021;27(3):520–8.
4. Flores E, Martínez-Racaj L, Torreblanca R, Blasco A, Lopez-Garrigós M, Gutiérrez I, et al. Clinical decision support system in laboratory medicine. Clin Chem Lab Med. 2024;62(7):1277–82.
5. Potočnik J, Foley S, Thomas E. Current and potential applications of artificial intelligence in medical imaging practice: a narrative review. J Med Imaging Radiat Sci. 2023;54(2):376–85.
6. Waqas A, Bui MM, Glassy EF, El Naqa I, Borkowski P, Borkowski AA, et al. Revolutionizing digital pathology with the power of generative artificial intelligence and foundation models. Lab Investig. 2023;103(11):100255.
7. Mennella C, Maniscalco U, De Pietro G, Esposito M. Ethical and regulatory challenges of AI technologies in healthcare: a narrative review. Heliyon. 2024;10(4):e26297.
8. Shortliffe E. Computer-based medical consultations: MYCIN. Elsevier; 2012.
9. Wraith SM, Aikins JS, Buchanan BG, Clancey WJ, Davis R, Fagan LM, et al. Computerized consultation system for selection of antimicrobial therapy. Am J Hosp Pharm. 1976;33(12):1304–8.
10. Delipetrev B, Tsinaraki, C. and Kostic, U. Historical evolution of artificial intelligence. Luxembourg: Publications Office of the European Union; 2020.
11. Kaul V, Enslin S, Gross SA. History of artificial intelligence in medicine. Gastrointest Endosc. 2020;92(4):807–12.
12. Davis R. Consultation, knowledge acquisition, and instruction: a case study. In: Chapter 3 in Szolovits P, editor. Artificial intelligence in medicine. Colorado: Westview Press; 1982. p. 57–78.
13. Yu VL, Buchanan BG, Shortliffe EH, Wraith SM, Davis R, Scott AC, et al. Evaluating the performance of a computer-based consultant. Comput Programs Biomed. 1979;9(1):95–102.
14. Yu VL, Fagan LM, Wraith SM, Clancey WJ, Scott AC, Hannigan J, et al. Antimicrobial selection by a computer: a blinded evaluation by infectious diseases experts. JAMA. 1979;242(12):1279–82.
15. Wallace W, Chan C, Chidambaram S, Hanna L, Iqbal FM, Acharya A, et al. The diagnostic and triage accuracy of digital and online symptom checker tools: a systematic review. NPJ Digit Med. 2022;5(1):118.
16. Semigran HL, Linder JA, Gidengil C, Mehrotra A. Evaluation of symptom checkers for self diagnosis and triage: audit study. BMJ. 2015;351:h3480.
17. Schmieding ML, Kopka M, Schmidt K, Schulz-Niethammer S, Balzer F, Feufel MA. Triage accuracy of symptom checker apps: 5-year follow-up evaluation. J Med Internet Res. 2022;24(5):e31810.
18. Bond WF, Schwartz LM, Weaver KR, Levick D, Giuliano M, Graber ML. Differential diagnosis generators: an evaluation of currently available computer programs. J Gen Intern Med. 2012;27(2):213–9.
19. Malik P, Pathania M, Rathaur VK. Overview of artificial intelligence in medicine. J Family Med Prim Care. 2019;8(7):2328–31.
20. Martinez-Franco AI, Sanchez-Mendiola M, Mazon-Ramirez JJ, Hernandez-Torres I, Rivero-Lopez C, Spicer T, et al. Diagnostic accuracy in Family Medicine residents using a clinical decision support system (DXplain): a randomized-controlled trial. Diagnosis (Berl). 2018;5(2):71–6.
21. Elkin PL, Liebow M, Bauer BA, Chaliki S, Wahner-Roedler D, Bundrick J, et al. The introduction of a diagnostic decision support system (DXplain™) into the workflow of a teaching hospital service can decrease the cost of service for diagnostically challenging Diagnostic Related Groups (DRGs). Int J Med Inform. 2010;79(11):772–7.
22. Kulikowski CA. Beginnings of artificial intelligence in medicine (AIM): computational artifice assisting scientific inquiry and clinical art – with reflections on present AIM challenges. Yearb Med Inform. 2019;28(1):249–56.
23. IBM Watson to Watsonx. Available from: https://www.ibm.com/watson.
24. Jie Z, Zhiying Z, Li L. A meta-analysis of Watson for Oncology in clinical application. Sci Rep. 2021;11(1):5792.
25. Tupasela A, Di Nucci E. Concordance as evidence in the Watson for Oncology decision-support system. AI & Soc. 2020;35(4):811–8.

26. Strickland E. IBM Watson, heal thyself: how IBM overpromised and underdelivered on AI health care. IEEE Spectr. 2019;56(4):24–31.
27. Muthukrishnan N, Maleki F, Ovens K, Reinhold C, Forghani B, Forghani R. Brief history of artificial intelligence. Neuroimaging Clin N Am. 2020;30(4):393–9.
28. Ren LY. Isabel Pro. J Can Health Libr Assoc/Journal de l'Association des bibliothèques de la santé du Canada. 2019;40(2):63–9.
29. Bridges JM. Computerized diagnostic decision support systems – a comparative performance study of Isabel Pro vs. ChatGPT4. Diagnosis. 2024;11:250.
30. Sibbald M, Monteiro S, Sherbino J, LoGiudice A, Friedman C, Norman G. Should electronic differential diagnosis support be used early or late in the diagnostic process? A multicentre experimental study of Isabel. BMJ Qual Saf. 2022;31(6):426–33.
31. Saab K, Tu T, Weng W-H, Tanno R, Stutz D, Wulczyn E, et al. Capabilities of Gemini models in medicine. arXiv preprint arXiv:240418416. 2024.
32. Angelov PP, Soares EA, Jiang R, Arnold NI, Atkinson PM. Explainable artificial intelligence: an analytical review. Wiley Interdiscip Rev Data Min Knowl Discov. 2021;11(5):e1424.
33. Meunier PY, Raynaud C, Guimaraes E, Gueyffier F, Letrilliart L. Barriers and facilitators to the use of clinical decision support systems in primary care: a mixed-methods systematic review. Ann Fam Med. 2023;21(1):57–69.

Overview of AI and Generative AI

4

Abstract

This chapter provides an overview of artificial intelligence, including generative artificial intelligence. The chapter simplifies the concepts underlying these technologies and clarifies their associated terminologies. The aim of this chapter is to build a foundation for understanding the role of artificial intelligence.

Keywords

Artificial Intelligence · Generative Artificial Intelligence · Machine Learning · Deep Learning · Large Language Models · Computational Reducibility · Information Processing · Transformer

4.1 Foundation of Information Processing

To effectively comprehend artificial intelligence and generative artificial intelligence, it is essential to establish a foundation in how information processing has evolved from traditional computing methods to sophisticated artificial intelligence-driven systems. The core concepts for traditional information processing, artificial intelligence, and generative artificial intelligence are outlined in Fig. 4.1 and Table 4.1.

4.1.1 Traditional Data Processing

Traditional computing relies on a straightforward, rule-based approach to processing data. Users define both the input data and the algorithms or mathematical formulas required to generate outputs. Computers execute the instructions sequentially to generate output, following a clearly predefined and unchanging logic.

T. Hirosawa, *Artificial Intelligence in Medical Diagnostics*,
https://doi.org/10.1007/978-981-95-4338-0_4

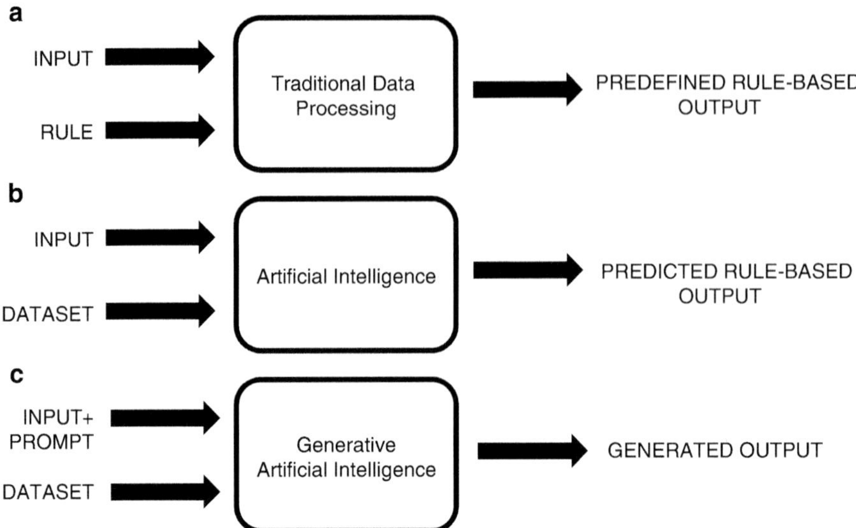

Fig. 4.1 Extremely simple concept of traditional information processing (**a**), artificial intelligence (**b**), and generative artificial intelligence (**c**)

An illustrative medical example of traditional processing is calculating corrected serum calcium levels using serum calcium and serum albumin concentrations. This calculation is a standard practice in clinical settings, as serum albumin directly affects measured calcium values. Users input the patient's serum calcium and serum albumin levels, and the computer applies the established formula: Corrected Calcium (mg/dL) = Measured Calcium + 0.8 × (4 − Serum Albumin). This method exemplifies traditional computing's reliance on explicitly programmed rules, fixed formulas, and predefined logic.

In traditional processing systems, the Central Processing Unit (CPU) predominates. CPUs are optimized for sequential processing, handling diverse operations like arithmetic calculations and logical evaluations efficiently.

However, traditional data processing exhibits significant limitations. It lacks adaptability when encountering data outside the predefined logic or when faced with complex interactions not captured by the provided algorithms. CPUs also face challenges processing highly parallel tasks efficiently, especially with large scales or unstructured data sets.

Despite these limitations, traditional data processing remains effective for routine, repetitive, and well-defined tasks. Its deterministic approach ensures reliability and consistency. Nonetheless, as data complexity increases and variable relationships grow more nuanced or unpredictable, traditional methods struggle to provide adequate solutions. This limitation highlights the necessity of advanced computational methodologies, notably those involving artificial intelligence. While traditional data processing is limited, artificial intelligence builds on these foundations to handle complexity and adapt to new information.

Table 4.1 Extremely simple concept of traditional information processing, artificial intelligence, and generative artificial intelligence

Section	Data processing	Suitable processor	Input	Information processing	Output	Strengths	Limitations	Example
4.1.1	Traditional data processing	Central Processing Unit	Input data	Pre-programmed rules/algorithms	Pre-defined results	Simple and reliable for routine tasks Easy to interpret and validate	Cannot adapt to new or unknown situations Requires explicit programming	Calculation Rule-based simple process
4.1.2	Artificial intelligence	Graphics Processing Unit	Input data	Learns rules from extensive dataset using algorithms	Predictions, classifications, decisions	Handles complex, unstructured, and large-scale data Learns patterns automatically	Needs large, diverse datasets to generalize well Limited interpretability (black box models)	Adaptable, can handle more complex tasks
4.1.3	Generative artificial intelligence	Graphics Processing Unit	Input data + prompt	Learns rules from extensive dataset using algorithms	Generated text, images, audio, movie	Creates novel solutions and outputs. Useful for tasks like content creation or augmentation	Computationally intensive. May generate inaccurate or biased content (e.g., hallucinations)	Creative, can generate novel outputs based on learned patterns

4.1.2 Data Processing in Artificial Intelligence

Artificial intelligence refers to a system's capability to perform cognitive functions traditionally associated with human intelligence, including learning, reasoning, interpreting, and interacting [1]. Unlike traditional computing, artificial intelligence systems do not rely solely on programmed rules but instead learn patterns directly from data. By identifying relationships in complex datasets, artificial intelligence models can inform predictions, guide decision-making, and support problem-solving across diverse applications [2].

Although terminology varies across disciplines, the lifecycle of artificial intelligence is commonly divided into two primary stages: the development (or training) phase and the deployment (or inference) phase [3, 4].

- Development Phase: In this stage, artificial intelligence models are trained on large datasets that contain examples of inputs and corresponding outputs. Through iterative optimization, the system learns to minimize errors by adjusting internal parameters. Depending on the approach, this may involve supervised learning (labeled datasets), unsupervised learning (unlabeled datasets), or reinforcement learning. Tasks in this phase include preprocessing data, feature extraction, model training, hyperparameter tuning, and performance evaluation on validation and test sets. For instance, in a clinical context, the inputs could consist of patient histories, laboratory results, and imaging findings, while outputs might correspond to disease classifications or prognostic outcomes.
- Deployment Phase: Once a model is sufficiently trained and validated, it enters the deployment phase. While often referred to as the "prediction phase," deployment encompasses far more than simply generating predictions. In this stage, the model is applied to new, unseen data, producing outputs that guide real-world decisions. Deployment also involves assessing model generalizability through independent validation sets, calibrating outputs for interpretability, monitoring performance over time, and addressing shifts in data distributions (so-called "dataset drift" or "concept drift"). In health-care settings, deployment may also include bias auditing, fairness assessments, regulatory compliance, and mechanisms for human oversight. Continuous monitoring ensures that the model remains reliable, safe, and ethically aligned as clinical environments evolve.

The distinctions between the development and deployment phases are summarized in Table 4.2.

Artificial intelligence effectively processes complex, high-dimensional, and unstructured data types, such as language, imaging, and health care-related data. Artificial intelligence can generalize predictions even to novel scenarios, enhancing its versatility. However, these capabilities require substantial computational resources. Artificial intelligence systems frequently depend on Graphics Processing Units (GPUs), specialized hardware optimized for parallel processing and necessary for machine learning's intensive computations [5].

Table 4.2 Key differences between development and deployment phases

Feature	Development phase	Deployment phase
Purpose	Train, optimize, and evaluate a model to minimize error and maximize performance	Apply the trained model to new data in real-world settings; ensure reliable, safe, and interpretable use
Data	Labeled data (supervised) or unlabeled data (unsupervised); typically split into training, validation, and test sets	New, unseen data from practice environments; may include continuously incoming data streams
Output	Trained model, tuned parameters, and performance metrics (e.g., accuracy, sensitivity, specificity)	Predictions, classifications, or decisions on new data; monitored results with potential for recalibration or retraining
Focus	Learning, optimization, error reduction, and model validation in controlled settings	Application, generalization, ongoing performance monitoring, calibration, fairness auditing, and adaptation to evolving conditions

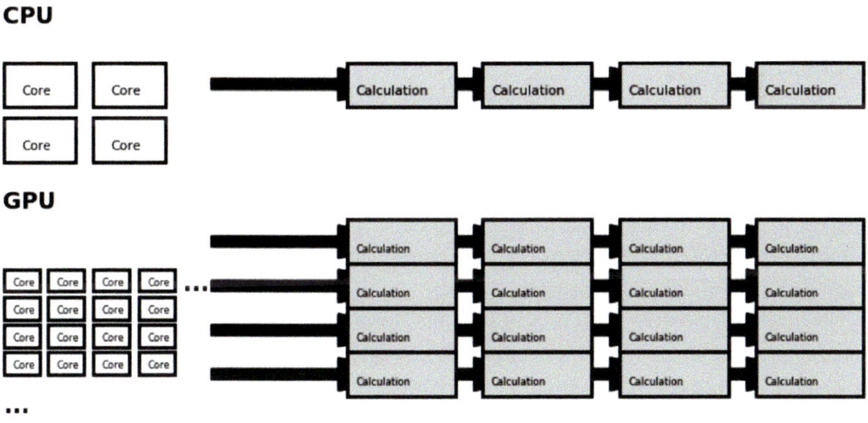

Fig. 4.2 Concept of architectural difference between Central Processing Unit (CPU) and Graphics Processing Unit (GPU)

GPUs were originally designed for graphics rendering but are uniquely suited for artificial intelligence tasks due to their ability to perform parallel computations rapidly. While CPUs execute operations sequentially, GPUs rise in importance, especially for handling the computational demands of training and validating complex models. The concept of architectural difference between CPU and GPU is shown in Fig. 4.2.

4.1.3 Data Processing in Generative Artificial Intelligence

Generative artificial intelligence is a specialized branch of artificial intelligence that moves beyond pattern recognition and predictive tasks to synthesize new data or content. These models are designed to synthesize information, allowing them to produce outputs that resemble human-created content. This ability to generate new and innovative outputs sets generative artificial intelligence apart from other artificial intelligence methods.

Generative artificial intelligence primarily relies on advanced neural network architectures, notably Generative Adversarial Networks (GANs) and transformer-based systems, such as GPT (Generative Pretrained Transformer) and DALL·E. These models undergo extensive training on large datasets to internalize inherent data patterns and subsequently generate contextually coherent outputs. For example, GANs synthesize medical images, whereas transformer-based models proficiently generate text with human-like coherence, facilitating tasks like summarization, translation, and reasoning.

The application scope of generative artificial intelligence extends beyond health care. In education, large language models have the potential to generate learning materials. Creative industries utilize generative artificial intelligence to produce scripts, music, and visual effects. In science and engineering, generative artificial intelligence models assist with simulation, design optimization, and the synthesis of novel molecular structures, significantly advancing research capabilities.

Generative artificial intelligence leverages extensive pretraining on diverse, unstructured datasets, coupled with fine-tuning for specific tasks. The pretraining phase imparts broad foundational knowledge, whereas fine-tuning tailors the learned information to specialized contexts, such as clinical data analysis or legal document generation. Attention mechanisms embedded within transformer architectures efficiently direct the model's focus toward critical data elements, enhancing both accuracy and computational efficiency.

Prior to generative artificial intelligence, human language was computationally irreducible due to its inherent complexity. Generative artificial intelligence models now make language "computationally reducible" [6], effectively translating intricate linguistic and conceptual patterns into computational processes. This reduction dramatically improves efficiency, accuracy, and feasibility for complex, real-time tasks.

Within medical applications, generative artificial intelligence facilitates automated generation of clinical documentation, diagnostic imaging interpretations, and drug discovery processes, offering significant clinical and research advancements [7, 8]. Nevertheless, generative artificial intelligence also poses substantial challenges, notably the potential generation of biased or inaccurate outputs, known as hallucinations. Addressing these challenges through rigorous validation, continuous monitoring, and ethical guidelines is critical for ensuring the safe and effective use of generative artificial intelligence in health care and beyond.

4.2 Terminology

Understanding key terminologies in artificial intelligence, including generative artificial intelligence, is crucial for navigating their applications. This section organizes the terminology into artificial intelligence and generative artificial intelligence.

4.2.1 Relationship Among Artificial Intelligence, Machine Learning, Deep Learning, Generative Artificial Intelligence, and Large Language Models

The relationship among artificial intelligence, machine learning, deep learning, generative artificial intelligence, and large language models is shown in Fig. 4.3.

4.2.2 Minimum Essential Terminology in Artificial Intelligence

- CPU (Central Processing Unit): The primary processor in a computer, handling general-purpose tasks.
- GPU (Graphics Processing Unit): A specialized processor optimized for parallel computation, essential for artificial intelligence model training due to its ability to handle large-scale computations efficiently [5].
- AI (Artificial Intelligence): The broader field focused on creating systems that can perform tasks requiring human-like intelligence, such as reasoning, learning, and decision-making.
- AGI (Artificial General Intelligence): A form of artificial intelligence capable of performing any intellectual task that a human can do. Unlike narrow artificial intelligence, which excels in specific domains, artificial general intelligence is designed to understand and reason across diverse tasks, adapting to new challenges without retraining. While theoretical at present, artificial general intelligence represents the ultimate goal for many researchers in the artificial intelligence field [9].
- Explainable AI (XAI): A branch of artificial intelligence focused on making models transparent (their inner workings are understandable) or interpretable (their decisions can be explained) [10]. Explainability is detailed in Chap. 11.

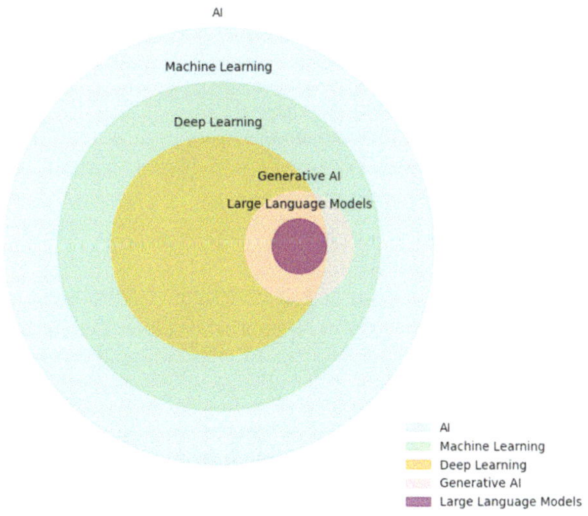

Fig. 4.3 Relationship among artificial intelligence, machine learning, deep learning, generative artificial intelligence, and large language models

- Edge computing: Edge computing is a distributed computing framework that brings computation and data storage closer to the location where it is needed [11]. Edge computing is detailed in Chap. 15.
- Standalone Artificial Intelligence: Standalone artificial intelligence refers to systems that operate independently without relying on continuous cloud connectivity.
- Edge Artificial Intelligence: This is a technical term that describes the location where artificial intelligence computation occurs. It specifically refers to artificial intelligence algorithms that are processed locally on a hardware device [12]. Edge artificial intelligence is also detailed in Chap. 15.
- Open-Source Artificial Intelligence Models: Systems characterized by their transparency and accessibility. The source code, training data, model architecture, and often the model weights are made publicly available. For generative artificial intelligence systems, openness is not an all-or-nothing feature. Openness is best understood as a composite and gradient notion [13].
- Closed Artificial Intelligence Models: The internal components, including code, data, and architecture, are kept confidential and are not shared publicly.
- Unimodal Artificial Intelligence Model: Artificial intelligence models designed to process only one type of data input. Also known as mono-modal or single-modal artificial intelligence, they are less complex but limited compared to multimodal systems.
- Multimodal Artificial Intelligence: Artificial intelligence models designed to process and integrate information from multiple types of data inputs, such as text, sound, image, and video [14].
- Machine Learning: A foundational artificial intelligence subfield focused on creating systems that learn and improve from experience without explicit programming.
- Deep Learning: A machine learning approach using neural networks with multiple layers to model complex data representations.
- Supervised Learning: Training models using labeled data, where input-output relationships are defined.
- Unsupervised Learning: Training models on unlabeled data to identify patterns or clusters.
- Neural Networks: Used synonymously with neural nets and artificial neural networks. Computational models inspired by the human brain, consisting of interconnected nodes organized into layers, namely input layer, hidden layer, and output layer, detailed in Fig. 4.4.
- Weights: The strength of connections between different neurons in the neural networks, detailed in Fig. 4.4.
- Convolutional Neural Network: One of the most common types of neural networks, which uses a specialized layer called a "convolutional layer" [15]. Typically contains massive hidden layers. This type is usually used for computer vision tasks [16].
- Hyperparameters: Parameters whose values are set before the learning process begins. They are not learned from datasets like model parameters, such as weights and biases in a neural network, but are defined by the user or determined

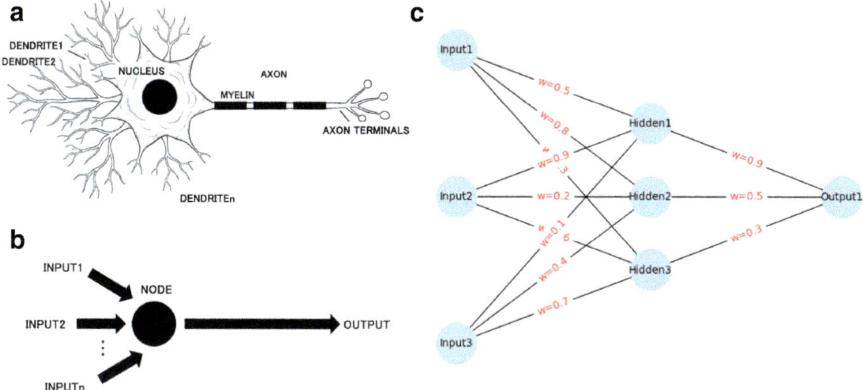

Fig. 4.4 The similarities between biological neurons (**a**) and artificial nodes in neural networks (**b**). Two-layered neural network with weights (**c**)

through experimentation. Examples of hyperparameters include learning rate, batch size, and number of epochs.

- TensorFlow and PyTorch: Popular open-source software libraries used for building and training artificial intelligence models, detailed in Chap. 2 [17, 18].
- Data augmentation: Technique used to artificially increase the size and diversity of your training dataset without collecting additional data.
- Application Programming Interface (API): A set of protocols and tools allowing different software applications to communicate with one another. APIs are crucial in integrating artificial intelligence systems into existing workflows and enabling seamless interaction between artificial intelligence tools and other software applications [19].

4.2.3 Minimum Essential Terminology in Generative Artificial Intelligence

- Generative Artificial Intelligence: A subset of artificial intelligence focused on generating new outputs, including text, images, audio, and video, based on patterns in the training data.
- Large Language Models (LLMs): Advanced artificial intelligence systems trained vast text datasets to understand and generate human-like language, such as GPT and LLaMA.
- Natural Language Processing (NLP): The artificial intelligence domain focused on understanding and generating human language.
- Tokenization: The process of breaking text or data into smaller units, referred to as tokens, for analysis by language models, detailed in Chap. 8.
- Prompt Engineering: The technique of designing input prompts to guide generative artificial intelligence models toward desired outputs [20].

- Zero-Shot Learning: The ability of an artificial intelligence model to perform tasks without prior training on the specific task [21, 22].
- One-Shot/Few-Shot Learning: The ability of artificial intelligence models to learn tasks from very limited examples, such as one example and few examples, respectively [23, 24].
- Chain of Thought: Technique to provide a series of intermediate reasoning steps before arriving at a final answer. It is a way to enhance the reasoning capabilities and improve the accuracy of LLMs, particularly for complex or multistep problems [25].
- Distillation: A technique for transferring knowledge from a large, complex model to a smaller, simpler model [26, 27]. The goal is to create a smaller model that retains much of the performance of the teacher but is more efficient in terms of memory footprint, computational cost, and inference speed.

In summary, this chapter explored the overview of artificial intelligence, including generative artificial intelligence, with foundational concepts, milestones, and advancements. These advancements highlight their transformative impact on various fields, particularly health care. While the potential for improving efficiency and creativity is extensive, challenges such as ethical considerations, data bias, and resource constraints must be addressed to ensure responsible and equitable adoption. Ultimately, generative artificial intelligence represents not just technological advancement, but paradigm shifts in how data is processed, synthesized, and utilized across disciplines. In the next chapter, we will explore the potential of artificial intelligence in medicine, especially medical diagnostics, highlighting how these advancements are made to revolutionize diagnostic accuracy, speed, and accessibility.

References

1. OECD. OECD science, technology and industry scoreboard 2017: the digital transformation 2017. Available from: https://www.oecd.org/en/publications/2017/11/oecd-science-technology-and-industry-scoreboard-2017_g1g74dc7.html.
2. Alaloul WS, Qureshi AH. Data processing using artificial neural networks. In: Dynamic data assimilation-beating the uncertainties. London: IntechOpen; 2020.
3. De Silva D, Alahakoon D. An artificial intelligence life cycle: from conception to production. Patterns. 2022;3(6):100489.
4. Desouza KC, Dawson GS, Chenok D. Designing, developing, and deploying artificial intelligence systems: lessons from and for the public sector. Bus Horiz. 2020;63(2):205–13.
5. Jeon W, Ko G, Lee J, Lee H, Ha D, Ro WW. Deep learning with GPUs. In: Advances in computers, vol. 122. Amsterdam: Elsevier; 2021. p. 167–215.
6. Wolfram S. What is ChatGPT doing: … and why does it work? Champaign, IL: Wolfram Media; 2023.
7. Liu J, Wang C, Liu S. Utility of ChatGPT in clinical practice. J Med Internet Res. 2023;25:e48568.
8. Sai S, Gaur A, Sai R, Chamola V, Guizani M, Rodrigues JJPC. Generative AI for transformative healthcare: a comprehensive study of emerging models, applications, case studies, and limitations. IEEE Access. 2024;12:31078–106.

9. Fahad M, Basri T, Hamza MA, Faisal S, Akbar A, Haider U, et al. The benefits and risks of artificial general intelligence (AGI). In: El Hajjami S, Kaushik K, Khan IU, editors. Artificial general intelligence (AGI) security: smart applications and sustainable technologies. Singapore: Springer Nature Singapore; 2025. p. 27–52.
10. Angelov PP, Soares EA, Jiang R, Arnold NI, Atkinson PM. Explainable artificial intelligence: an analytical review. WIREs Data Min Knowl Discov. 2021;11(5):e1424.
11. Khan WZ, Ahmed E, Hakak S, Yaqoob I, Ahmed A. Edge computing: a survey. Futur Gener Comput Syst. 2019;97:219–35.
12. Singh R, Gill SS. Edge AI: a survey. Internet Things Cyber-Phys Syst. 2023;3:71–92.
13. Liesenfeld A, Dingemanse M. Rethinking open source generative AI: open washing and the EU AI Act. In: Proceedings of the 2024 ACM conference on fairness, accountability, and transparency. Rio de Janeiro: Association for Computing Machinery; 2024. p. 1774–87.
14. Acosta JN, Falcone GJ, Rajpurkar P, Topol EJ. Multimodal biomedical AI. Nat Med. 2022;28(9):1773–84.
15. Abiodun OI, Jantan A, Omolara AE, Dada KV, Mohamed NA, Arshad H. State-of-the-art in artificial neural network applications: a survey. Heliyon. 2018;4(11):e00938.
16. Santos CFGD, Papa JP. Avoiding overfitting: a survey on regularization methods for convolutional neural networks. ACM Comput Surv. 2022;54(10s):Article 213.
17. Abadi M, Barham P, Chen J, Chen Z, Davis A, Dean J, et al., editors. TensorFlow: a system for large-scale machine learning. 12th USENIX symposium on operating systems design and implementation (OSDI 16). Berkeley, CA: USENIX Association; 2016.
18. Paszke A. Pytorch: an imperative style, high-performance deep learning library. arXiv preprint arXiv:191201703. 2019.
19. Ofoeda J, Boateng R, Effah J. Application programming interface (API) research: a review of the past to inform the future. Int J Enterp Inf Syst. 2019;15(3):76–95.
20. Zaghir J, Naguib M, Bjelogrlic M, Névéol A, Tannier X, Lovis C. Prompt engineering paradigms for medical applications: scoping review. J Med Internet Res. 2024;26:e60501.
21. Palatucci M, Pomerleau D, Hinton GE, Mitchell TM. Zero-shot learning with semantic output codes. Adv Neural Inf Process Syst. 2009;22:1410–18.
22. Socher R, Ganjoo M, Manning CD, Ng A. Zero-shot learning through cross-modal transfer. Adv Neural Inf Proces Syst. 2013;26:1410–18.
23. Brown T, Mann B, Ryder N, Subbiah M, Kaplan JD, Dhariwal P, et al. Language models are few-shot learners. Adv Neural Inf Proces Syst. 2020;33:1877–901.
24. Vinyals O, Blundell C, Lillicrap T, Wierstra D. Matching networks for one shot learning. Adv Neural Inf Process Syst. 2016;29:1410–18.
25. Wei J, Wang X, Schuurmans D, Bosma M, Xia F, Chi E, et al. Chain-of-thought prompting elicits reasoning in large language models. Adv Neural Inf Process Syst. 2022;35:24824–37.
26. Yu R, Liu S, Wang X. Dataset distillation: a comprehensive review. IEEE Trans Pattern Anal Mach Intell. 2024;46(1):150–70. https://doi.org/10.1109/TPAMI.2023.3323376.
27. Guo D, Yang D, Zhang H, Song J, Zhang R, Xu R, et al. DeepSeek-R1: incentivizing reasoning capability in LLMs via reinforcement learning. arXiv preprint arXiv:250112948. 2025.

The Potential of AI in Diagnostics

5

Abstract

This chapter explores the transformative role of artificial intelligence in the field of medicine, especially medical diagnostics, emphasizing its potential to revolutionize traditional diagnostic practices. It discusses the significant bottlenecks in existing systems, including clinical reasoning, teamwork, communication, diagnostic test usage, and health information technology. This chapter also explores how artificial intelligence addresses these challenges. These innovations collectively highlight the capacity of artificial intelligence to elevate diagnostic precision and accessibility while mitigating long-standing challenges. The chapter further examines the emerging role of generative artificial intelligence, focusing on its advantages, risks, and the strategies needed for effective integration into clinical workflows. By highlighting real-world applications and potential pitfalls, the chapter sets the stage for understanding how artificial intelligence can collaborate with health-care professionals to enhance medical diagnostics.

Keywords

Clinical reasoning · Diagnostic bottlenecks · Health information technology · Communication in healthcare · Teamwork in diagnostics · Diagnostic test utilization

5.1 Representative Artificial Intelligence in Medicine

5.1.1 Artificial Intelligence in Medicine

The integration of artificial intelligence into medicine represents one of the most transformative developments in modern health care [1, 2]. Artificial intelligence has the potential to address long-standing challenges, improve patient outcomes, and enhance the efficiency of health care delivery. By leveraging large datasets, machine

T. Hirosawa, *Artificial Intelligence in Medical Diagnostics*,
https://doi.org/10.1007/978-981-95-4338-0_5

learning models can identify patterns, generate predictions, and provide actionable insights that would be difficult or impossible for humans to discern.

In medicine, artificial intelligence has found applications in diverse areas, including diagnostics, personalized medicine, drug discovery, and operational efficiency:

- Diagnostics: Artificial intelligence algorithms analyze complex medical data, such as imaging studies, laboratory results, and even genomic information, to detect diseases earlier and with precision. For example, artificial intelligence-powered tools assist radiologists in identifying subtle abnormalities on X-rays or computed tomography scans that might be overlooked during manual review [3].
- Personalized Medicine: Artificial intelligence enables health-care professionals to tailor treatments based on individual patient characteristics, such as genetic profiles or response to previous therapies. This approach is central to precision medicine, which aims to optimize therapeutic outcomes for each patient [4].
- Drug Discovery: Machine learning accelerates the drug development process by predicting the efficacy of compounds, identifying potential side effects, and modeling complex molecular interactions [5]. A groundbreaking example is AlphaFold, which has revolutionized the field of structural biology by predicting protein folding with remarkable accuracy [6]. This breakthrough facilitates the identification of new drug targets and the design of novel therapeutics, significantly reducing the timeline and cost of drug discovery.
- Operational Efficiency: Artificial intelligence streamlines administrative tasks, such as scheduling, billing, and resource allocation, freeing up health-care professionals to focus more on patient care.

Artificial intelligence's potential in medicine is not without challenges. Ethical considerations, data privacy, and the need for transparent and explainable artificial intelligence systems remain critical areas of focus. Despite these hurdles, the integration of artificial intelligence is fundamentally reshaping health care, enabling more accurate, efficient, and equitable medical practices.

5.1.2 Artificial Intelligence in Diagnosis

Artificial intelligence has had a profound impact on medical diagnostics, transforming how diseases are detected, monitored, and treated. By automating and enhancing the diagnostic process, artificial intelligence-powered tools have improved both the accuracy and speed of diagnosis, addressing key pain points in traditional diagnostic methods.

Artificial intelligence in diagnosis operates across multiple modalities:

- Clinical Reasoning including Differential-Diagnosis: Artificial intelligence systems enhance clinical reasoning by integrating patient history, symptoms, and investigation results to generate differential diagnoses. For example, artificial intelligence tools like Isabel Pro have been successfully implemented to assist health-care professionals by providing ranked lists of potential conditions based on input patient data [7]. These systems help health-care professionals broaden differential diagnoses and validate initial impressions, ensuring a comprehensive approach to patient care. Therefore, tools such as diagnostic decision support systems assist health-care professionals in systematically expanding differential diagnoses and narrowing down differential diagnoses, improving diagnostic accuracy and efficiency.

- Medical Imaging: Artificial intelligence models trained on vast datasets of medical images, such as X-rays, computed tomography scans, and magnetic resonance imaging, can identify abnormalities like tumors, fractures, and vascularity [8]. For instance, artificial intelligence algorithms have demonstrated the ability to detect lung nodules on chest computed tomography scans with accuracy comparable to that of experienced radiologists [9].
- Laboratory Diagnostics: Artificial intelligence systems analyze laboratory test results, flagging anomalies that may indicate underlying conditions. By identifying patterns across multiple parameters, artificial intelligence tools provide a comprehensive view of a patient's health status [10].
- Genomics and Pathology: In fields like genomics, artificial intelligence aids in identifying genetic mutations associated with diseases, while in pathology, it analyzes digitized tissue samples to detect cancerous cells or classify tumors [11, 12].
- Point-of-Care Devices: Artificial intelligence is increasingly integrated into wearable and handheld diagnostic tools, such as portable ultrasound devices and smartwatches. These tools empower health-care professionals to perform real-time diagnostics at the bedside or in remote locations, improving accessibility to care [13].

The success of artificial intelligence in diagnostics can be attributed to its ability to process large, complex datasets with unparalleled speed and accuracy. However, challenges remain, including the need for robust validation, integration into existing health-care systems, and addressing ethical concerns such as bias and transparency. As artificial intelligence continues to evolve, its role in diagnostics will expand, driving advancements in precision medicine and ultimately improving patient outcomes.

5.2 Bottlenecks in Traditional Diagnostics

This section introduces the diagnostic process and emphasizes its critical role in health care. Traditional diagnostic systems face notable challenges and bottlenecks that impede efficiency and accuracy. According to the Committee on Diagnostic Error in Health Care, health-care professional certification and accreditation organizations must ensure that practitioners maintain essential competencies required for effective diagnostic performance. These competencies include clinical reasoning;

teamwork; effective communication with patients, families, and colleagues; proper use and interpretation of diagnostic tests; and adeptness in health information technology [14].

To uphold these competencies, regular assessments, targeted training programs, and continuous educational initiatives are recommended. However, the implementation of these recommendations encounters several challenges, including inconsistent access to resources, varying standards across different health-care settings, and disparities in training opportunities among institutions. Table 5.1 summarizes the bottlenecks present in traditional medical diagnostics and potential resolutions utilizing artificial intelligence, generative artificial intelligence, and unspecialized generative artificial intelligence.

5.2.1 Bottlenecks in Clinical Reasoning

Clinical reasoning presents a fundamental challenge due to its reliance on integrating complex information within restrictive time and resource constraints. Diagnostic errors often occur due to limitations in interpreting data, cognitive biases, or subjective judgments, even among experienced health-care professionals. Such limitations significantly affect diagnostic accuracy, leading to misdiagnosis and delayed treatments, adversely impacting patient outcomes.

Table 5.1 Bottlenecks in medical diagnostics and potential resolution with artificial intelligence (AI), generative AI, and unspecialized generative AI

Bottlenecks	Resolving with AI	Resolving with generative AI	Resolving with unspecialized generative AI
Clinical reasoning	Provides decision-support tools to analyze datasets and reduce cognitive biases	Generates synthetic datasets for training AI models to handle complex scenarios	Provides preliminary diagnostic insights using generalized data patterns
Teamwork	Facilitates collaboration through centralized platforms for real-time data sharing	Creates shared visualizations of workflows to align team strategies	Improves access in resource-limited settings but lacks domain-specific adjustments
Communication	Simplifies complex information into comprehensible summaries for all stakeholders	Enhances clarity using NLP to simplify complex medical findings	Generates diagnostic summaries that may be overly technical or unclear
Diagnostic test usage	Assists in selecting relevant tests and integrating findings into actionable insights	Simulates test outcomes under diverse scenarios to optimize selection	Identifies patterns or anomalies but may misinterpret specific contexts
Health information technology	Streamlines data integration and improves interoperability	Harmonizes disparate data systems for cohesive operation	Offers accessible but less reliable tools for underserved regions

5.2.2 Bottlenecks in Teamwork

Teamwork bottlenecks exacerbate challenges in traditional diagnostics, as successful diagnosis depends heavily on seamless collaboration among diverse health-care professionals. Fragmented communication within teams can result in incomplete information exchanges, poor coordination, and critical insights being overlooked. Moreover, the absence of standardized communication protocols further complicates team interactions, severely impairing the diagnostic process and obstructing the delivery of optimal patient care.

5.2.3 Bottlenecks in Communication

Communication issues introduce additional complexity into the diagnostic process, particularly affecting interactions between health-care professionals and patients. Many patients struggle to comprehend medical terminology or the implications of diagnostic outcomes, which lead to misunderstandings and confusion regarding their health conditions. This issue is further aggravated by inadequate communication skills among some health-care professionals, contributing to unclear treatment plans and insufficient follow-up care. Additionally, as detailed previously in Sect. 5.2.2, failures in communication among health-care professionals themselves, stemming from fragmented information sharing and inconsistent documentation practices, severely impact diagnostic accuracy and patient safety. Addressing these communication bottlenecks requires improved training, effective patient education strategies, and standardized protocols for professional exchanges to minimize diagnostic errors and delays [15].

5.2.4 Bottlenecks in Diagnostic Tests

The appropriate use of diagnostic tests, along with the effective interpretation and application of their results, presents a significant bottleneck. Overreliance on specific tests, misinterpretation of results, or failure to integrate diagnostic results into clear, actionable plans can substantially delay or diminish diagnostic accuracy. These issues are often compounded by fragmented individual efforts, departmental workflows, and institutional processes, contributing to system overload and significant logistical barriers [14].

5.2.5 Bottlenecks in Health Information Technology

Health information technology, intended to enhance diagnostic processes, frequently becomes a bottleneck due to systemic inefficiencies, interoperability issues, or user-related errors. Many technological platforms lack seamless integration, adding unnecessary complexity and slowing diagnostic workflows. Furthermore, disparities in access to health technology, particularly in remote or underserved regions, intensify health inequities and delay essential care, adversely affecting vulnerable patient populations.

5.3 Resolving Diagnostic Bottlenecks with Artificial Intelligence

This section explores the core benefits of artificial intelligence in addressing key bottlenecks identified in clinical reasoning, teamwork, and communication within diagnostics.

5.3.1 Artificial Intelligence for Clinical Reasoning

Artificial intelligence enhances clinical reasoning by providing decision-support tools that analyze large datasets and suggest potential diagnoses based on evidence. Machine learning algorithms can mitigate cognitive biases and highlight hidden patterns not apparent to health-care professionals. By integrating these tools into diagnostic workflows, health-care professionals can make more informed and timely decisions, reducing errors and delays.

For example, an artificial intelligence-powered diagnostic support tool can analyze a complex patient presentation—such as multiple symptoms of autoimmune disease and infection—and generate a ranked list of possible differential diagnoses. Evidence shows that electronic differential diagnostic support systems can expand diagnostic hypotheses and improve accuracy. Importantly, it also increased the likelihood of including the correct diagnosis in the differential by about 7–8%, regardless of experience level [7].

5.3.2 Artificial Intelligence for Teamwork

In diagnostic teamwork, artificial intelligence fosters collaboration by creating centralized platforms for sharing diagnostic insights and patient data among health-care professionals. These systems improve coordination and ensure that all team members have access to the same information in real-time. Such advancements reduce fragmentation within teams and streamline diagnostic processes. In intensive care units, for instance, artificial intelligence-driven dashboards can visualize a patient's trajectory—including vitals, lab trends, and medication responses—enabling physicians, nurses, and pharmacists to coordinate care more effectively [16].

5.3.3 Artificial Intelligence for Communication

Effective communication with patients and health-care teams is further strengthened through artificial intelligence-driven interfaces that simplify the explanation of complex medical findings. Artificial intelligence-driven tools can translate diagnostic results into comprehensible summaries for patients, while also aiding interprofessional communication by standardizing terminology and improving clarity. For example, an artificial intelligence software embedded in electronic health records can generate plain-language explanations of investigation results for patients [17].

5.3.4 Artificial Intelligence for Diagnostic Tests

This section focuses on how artificial intelligence addresses challenges in the appropriate use of diagnostic tests and the application of results in clinical decision-making. Artificial intelligence assists health-care professionals in selecting the most relevant diagnostic tests for specific conditions by analyzing patient history, symptoms, and existing data. Decision-support systems reduce overreliance on unnecessary tests, minimizing health-care costs and improving efficiency. Once results are available, artificial intelligence tools integrate findings into actionable insights, suggesting follow-up investigations or treatment plans tailored to the patient's needs.

For instance, artificial intelligence-powered platforms can prioritize critical test results, ensuring prompt attention to urgent cases. They also enable more accurate interpretation of complex results, such as genomic or imaging data, by identifying subtle patterns that may be missed by health-care professionals. This ensures that diagnostic test usage is both effective and aligned with clinical goals.

5.3.5 Artificial Intelligence for Health Information Technology

Artificial intelligence offers practical solutions to address bottlenecks in health information technology systems, including inefficiencies, interoperability issues, and user-related challenges. One key improvement is the use of artificial intelligence to streamline data integration from multiple sources, ensuring compatibility with electronic health records. This reduces fragmentation and simplifies access to comprehensive patient data. Artificial intelligence also enhances interoperability by converting disparate data formats into standardized outputs, enabling seamless communication between different health-care systems.

To address user challenges, artificial intelligence-driven interfaces prioritize ease of access by automating routine tasks and reducing the cognitive load on health-care professionals. For example, predictive analytics tools can identify patterns in patient data, providing actionable insights without requiring manual analysis. Continuous monitoring and adaptive learning further ensure that artificial intelligence systems remain responsive to user needs and system updates, maintaining efficiency over time. Beyond addressing individual bottlenecks, artificial intelligence must also be integrated effectively with existing workflows.

5.3.6 Strategies for Integration and Adoption

Explores the methods for harmonizing artificial intelligence with current diagnostic workflows and technologies, emphasizing a balanced approach between innovation and practical application [18]. One approach involves hybrid diagnostic models that combine artificial intelligence-generated insights with traditional diagnostic techniques, enhancing the accuracy and reliability of results while preserving health-care professional oversight. Another significant focus is overcoming integration challenges, which includes addressing technical hurdles like data interoperability, infrastructural limitations, and human factors such as resistance to adopting new technologies. Furthermore, ensuring compatibility and interoperability with existing systems, particularly electronic health records, is critical. This compatibility enables seamless data exchange and collaboration between artificial intelligence systems and health-care professionals, enhancing workflow efficiency [19].

5.4 Generative Artificial Intelligence to Resolve Diagnostic Bottlenecks

Generative artificial intelligence addresses multiple critical diagnostic challenges by improving clinical reasoning, fostering effective teamwork, streamlining communication, optimizing diagnostic test utilization, and resolving barriers inherent in health information technology systems [20]. Unlike conventional models that only classify or predict, generative models simulate and expand clinical scenarios, thereby addressing gaps and enhancing diagnostic capacity.

5.4.1 Generative Artificial Intelligence for Clinical Reasoning

Generative artificial intelligence can enhance clinical reasoning in two key ways. First, it can generate synthetic datasets of medical data designed to replicate complex diagnostic scenarios that health-care professionals encounter in real-world practice. These datasets are particularly useful in training artificial intelligence models to recognize rare medical conditions or atypical presentations—cases that deviate from typical symptoms or diagnostic patterns. By leveraging such diverse datasets, generative artificial intelligence equips diagnostic tools to handle a broader spectrum of clinical situations, thereby reducing diagnostic errors and enhancing decision-making accuracy in clinical practice [21].

Second, these models can directly assist health-care professionals by analyzing complex cases and suggesting potential diagnoses. Studies have shown that large language models like GPT can achieve high accuracy in suggesting potential diagnoses from complex case reports, sometimes on par with human health-care professionals [22, 23].

5.4.2 Generative Artificial Intelligence for Teamwork

In teamwork, generative artificial intelligence facilitates collaboration among health-care professionals by generating clear, shared visualizations of patient data and diagnostic processes. These visualizations translate complex medical information into intuitive graphics or diagrams, which assist health-care teams in aligning their diagnostic strategies, improving understanding of patient cases, and reducing the likelihood of misinterpretations or communication errors.

For instance, generative artificial intelligence can create detailed 3D models of human anatomy, allowing medical students and surgical teams to visualize and practice complex procedures in a simulated environment without risk to patients [24]. This shared understanding is critical for effective collaboration and decision-making in multidisciplinary teams.

5.4.3 Generative Artificial Intelligence for Communication

Communication improvements are a substantial benefit of generative artificial intelligence. It can convert specialized medical terminology, often referred to as medical jargon, into easily understandable summaries for patients, thereby enhancing patient engagement and adherence to medical recommendations. Research revealed that a large language model could transform technical hospital discharge summaries into a patient-friendly format [25]. Simultaneously, it provides precise, yet succinct clinical reports tailored for health-care professionals, thus ensuring clarity, efficiency, and accuracy in diagnostic information sharing [26].

5.4.4 Generative Artificial Intelligence for Diagnostic Tests

Generative artificial intelligence optimizes diagnostic test usage by simulating test results across various hypothetical patient scenarios. These simulations enable health-care professionals to predict the most effective tests for specific conditions, optimizing resource use and patient management strategies. Additionally, generative artificial intelligence serves a crucial role in the validation of artificial intelligence-driven diagnostic tools, rigorously assessing their reliability and robustness through diverse, synthetic scenarios before real-world application. In medical imaging, generative artificial intelligence can enhance the quality of low resolution scans, making them clearer for radiologists [27].

5.4.5 Generative Artificial Intelligence for Health Information Technology

Health information technology bottlenecks—challenges associated with managing and integrating disparate medical data systems—are effectively addressed through generative artificial intelligence's capability to standardize diverse data formats and intelligently fill in gaps within incomplete datasets. By harmonizing incompatible data systems, generative artificial intelligence ensures seamless interoperability, facilitating efficient integration of various diagnostic platforms into unified health-care information technology ecosystems. For instance, artificial intelligence-powered tools that listen to and document patient encounters in real-time can generate draft clinical notes, reducing the administrative burden on health-care professionals [28]. This integration mitigates workflow interruptions due to technical constraints and promotes smoother diagnostic operations across health-care facilities.

5.5 The Potential of Unspecialized or Untrained Generative AI in Medical Diagnostics

While generative artificial intelligence has shown immense potential in advancing medical diagnostics, the use of unspecialized or untrained generative artificial intelligence systems presents both opportunities and challenges [29]. Unlike artificial intelligence systems tailored specifically for health care, unspecialized generative artificial intelligence lacks medical training. However, these systems can still provide valuable diagnostic assistance in specific contexts.

5.5.1 Advantages of Unspecialized Generative Artificial Intelligence

One notable advantage of unspecialized generative artificial intelligence is its ability to deliver certain diagnostic performance levels even without specific training, as detailed in Chap. 9. These systems can process large volumes of generalized data to cover various domains. For example, GPT-3, developed by OpenAI, has been trained on several major data sources, including Common Crawl and English-language Wikipedia [30]. These data sources contain not only general information but also science and medicine [31, 32]. These capabilities make GPT-3 accessible tools for preliminary diagnostics or in situations where access to specialized health-care resources is limited. It is important to note that the GPT-3 model has since been retired. It has been replaced by more advanced iterations that address prior limitations and further enhance diagnostic accuracy and applicability. These new models continue to build on GPT-3's foundation while offering improved functionality tailored to evolving needs.

Large language model-based systems, such as Google's Articulate Medical Intelligence Explorer (AMIE), have demonstrated promising diagnostic performance even before specialized training. In a recent study without review processing, the artificial intelligence system exhibited standalone performance that exceeded that of unassisted health-care professionals, achieving a top 10 differential accuracy of 59% compared to 34% ($p = 0.04$). Additionally, health-care professionals assisted by AMIE generated more comprehensive differential lists and achieved higher diagnostic accuracy than those without artificial intelligence assistance [33]. Such findings highlight the potential of unspecialized generative artificial intelligence to augment clinical decision-making effectively.

Another significant benefit is their accessibility. Unspecialized generative artificial intelligence systems are often widely available and cost-effective, making them viable options for resource-limited settings or as supplementary tools in overstretched health-care systems. This accessibility can help bridge gaps in health-care delivery, especially in underserved regions.

5.5.2 Risks and Challenges of Unspecialized Generative Artificial Intelligence

Despite these advantages, there are risks associated with relying on these systems for critical decision-making, as detailed in Chap. 10. Generative artificial intelligence models trained on generalized data may produce inaccurate or misleading diagnostic suggestions, lacking the specificity required for medical contexts. Additionally, these systems often fail to account for the nuances of clinical reasoning and the context-sensitive nature of diagnostics.

Communication challenges also remain a concern. Unspecialized generative artificial intelligence may generate explanations or diagnostic summaries that are unclear, overly technical, or incorrect, further complicating interactions between health-care professionals and patients. Such issues can erode trust and hinder effective decision-making.

5.5.3 Integration and Mitigation Strategies

The integration of unspecialized generative artificial intelligence into health-care workflows necessitates caution. Without proper validation and oversight, these systems could introduce errors, disrupt teamwork by providing inconsistent information, and fail to align with health information technology systems effectively. To mitigate these risks, it is essential to supplement their use with expert oversight and to ensure they operate within clearly defined parameters.

To maximize the benefits while addressing the risks, generative artificial intelligence systems should be rigorously trained on high-quality, domain-specific data whenever possible. Robust governance frameworks and validation processes are crucial to ensuring these tools meet the highest standards of reliability, accuracy, and ethical responsibility in medical diagnostics.

In conclusion, this chapter highlights the potential of artificial intelligence to transform medical diagnostics by addressing key bottlenecks and enabling more efficient, accurate, and accessible health-care solutions. While the advantages of artificial intelligence, including generative artificial intelligence systems, are vast, careful implementation and validation remain essential to mitigate risks and ensure ethical, patient-centered care. This involves rigorously testing artificial intelligence systems across diverse scenarios, ensuring transparency in decision-making processes, and validating outputs through clinical trials. Additionally, establishing clear guidelines and governance frameworks ensures that artificial intelligence tools are integrated responsibly and align with the broader goals of patient safety and care quality. As the next chapter explores collaboration between artificial intelligence developers and health-care professionals, it becomes evident that fostering effective partnerships is critical to fully realizing artificial intelligence's potential in diagnostics and beyond.

References

1. Bajwa J, Munir U, Nori A, Williams B. Artificial intelligence in healthcare: transforming the practice of medicine. Future Healthc J. 2021;8(2):e188–e94.
2. Malik P, Pathania M, Rathaur VK. Overview of artificial intelligence in medicine. J Family Med Prim Care. 2019;8(7):2328–31.
3. Kelly BS, Judge C, Bollard SM, Clifford SM, Healy GM, Aziz A, et al. Radiology artificial intelligence: a systematic review and evaluation of methods (RAISE). Eur Radiol. 2022;32(11):7998–8007.
4. Quazi S. Artificial intelligence and machine learning in precision and genomic medicine. Med Oncol. 2022;39(8):120.
5. Huang P-S, Boyken SE, Baker D. The coming of age of de novo protein design. Nature. 2016;537(7620):320–7.
6. Abramson J, Adler J, Dunger J, Evans R, Green T, Pritzel A, et al. Accurate structure prediction of biomolecular interactions with AlphaFold 3. Nature. 2024;630(8016):493–500.
7. Sibbald M, Monteiro S, Sherbino J, LoGiudice A, Friedman C, Norman G. Should electronic differential diagnosis support be used early or late in the diagnostic process? A multicentre experimental study of Isabel. BMJ Qual Saf. 2022;31(6):426–33.
8. Anwar SM, Majid M, Qayyum A, Awais M, Alnowami M, Khan MK. Medical image analysis using convolutional neural networks: a review. J Med Syst. 2018;42(11):226.
9. Potočnik J, Foley S, Thomas E. Current and potential applications of artificial intelligence in medical imaging practice: a narrative review. J Med Imaging Radiat Sci. 2023;54(2):376–85.
10. Yang HS, Wang F, Greenblatt MB, Huang SX, Zhang Y. AI chatbots in clinical laboratory medicine: foundations and trends. Clin Chem. 2023;69(11):1238–46.
11. Waqas A, Bui MM, Glassy EF, El Naqa I, Borkowski P, Borkowski AA, et al. Revolutionizing digital pathology with the power of generative artificial intelligence and foundation models. Lab Investig. 2023;103(11):100255.
12. Dias R, Torkamani A. Artificial intelligence in clinical and genomic diagnostics. Genome Med. 2019;11(1):70.
13. Lilly CM, Soni AV, Dunlap D, Hafer N, Picard MA, Buchholz B, et al. Advancing point-of-care testing by application of machine learning techniques and artificial intelligence. Chest. 2025;167(1):152–9.
14. Balogh EP, Miller BT, Ball JR. Improving diagnosis in health care. Washington, DC: National Academies Press; 2015.
15. Dingley C, Daugherty K, Derieg MK, Persing R. Advances in patient safety Improving patient safety through provider communication strategy enhancements. In: Henriksen K, Battles JB, Keyes MA, Grady ML, editors. Advances in patient safety: new directions and alternative approaches (vol 3: performance and tools). Rockville: Agency for Healthcare Research and Quality (US); 2008.
16. Godbole AA, Paras, Mehra M, Banerjee S, Roy P, Deb N, et al. Enhancing infection control in ICUS through AI: a literature review. Health Sci Rep. 2025;8(1):e70288.

17. Bala S, Keniston A, Burden M. Patient perception of plain-language medical notes generated using artificial intelligence software: pilot mixed-methods study. JMIR Form Res. 2020;4(6):e16670.
18. Muthukrishnan N, Maleki F, Ovens K, Reinhold C, Forghani B, Forghani R. Brief history of artificial intelligence. Neuroimaging Clin N Am. 2020;30(4):393–9.
19. Alowais SA, Alghamdi SS, Alsuhebany N, Alqahtani T, Alshaya AI, Almohareb SN, et al. Revolutionizing healthcare: the role of artificial intelligence in clinical practice. BMC Med Educ. 2023;23(1):689.
20. Liu J, Wang C, Liu S. Utility of ChatGPT in clinical practice. J Med Internet Res. 2023;25:e48568.
21. Takita H, Kabata D, Walston SL, Tatekawa H, Saito K, Tsujimoto Y, et al. A systematic review and meta-analysis of diagnostic performance comparison between generative AI and physicians. NPJ Digit Med. 2025;8(1):175.
22. Hirosawa T, Harada Y, Mizuta K, Sakamoto T, Tokumasu K, Shimizu T. Diagnostic performance of generative artificial intelligences for a series of complex case reports. Digit Health. 2024;10:20552076241265215.
23. Cabral S, Restrepo D, Kanjee Z, Wilson P, Crowe B, Abdulnour R-E, et al. Clinical reasoning of a generative artificial intelligence model compared with physicians. JAMA Intern Med. 2024;184(5):581–3.
24. Lee J-O, Zhou H-Y, Berzin TM, Sodickson DK, Rajpurkar P. Multimodal generative AI for interpreting 3D medical images and videos. NPJ Digit Med. 2025;8(1):273.
25. Zaretsky J, Kim JM, Baskharoun S, Zhao Y, Austrian J, Aphinyanaphongs Y, et al. Generative artificial intelligence to transform inpatient discharge summaries to patient-friendly language and format. JAMA Netw Open. 2024;7(3):e240357-e.
26. Rubinstein B, Matos S. Value creation for healthcare ecosystems through artificial intelligence applied to physician-to-physician communication: a systematic review. Neural Process Lett. 2025;57(1):6.
27. Kim W, Jeon S-Y, Byun G, Yoo H, Choi J-H. A systematic review of deep learning-based denoising for low-dose computed tomography from a perceptual quality perspective. Biomed Eng Lett. 2024;14(6):1153–73.
28. Leung TI, Coristine AJ, Benis A. AI scribes in health care: balancing transformative potential with responsible integration. JMIR Med Inform. 2025;13:e80898.
29. Sai S, Gaur A, Sai R, Chamola V, Guizani M, Rodrigues JJPC. Generative AI for transformative healthcare: a comprehensive study of emerging models, applications, case studies, and limitations. IEEE Access. 2024;12:31078–106.
30. Brown T, Mann B, Ryder N, Subbiah M, Kaplan JD, Dhariwal P, et al. Language models are few-shot learners. Adv Neural Inf Process Syst. 2020;33:1877–901.
31. Dodge J, Sap M, Marasović A, Agnew W, Ilharco G, Groeneveld D, et al. Documenting large webtext corpora: a case study on the colossal clean crawled corpus. arXiv preprint arXiv:210408758. 2021.
32. Heilman JM, West AG. Wikipedia and medicine: quantifying readership, editors, and the significance of natural language. J Med Internet Res. 2015;17(3):e62.
33. Karthikesalingam A, Natarajan P. AMIE: a research AI system for diagnostic medical reasoning and conversations [Internet]. 2024. [2/22/2025]. Available from: https://research.google/blog/amie-a-research-ai-system-for-diagnostic-medical-reasoning-and-conversations/.

Bridging the Gap: Collaboration Between AI Developers and Health-Care Professionals

6

Abstract

The integration of artificial intelligence into health care has the potential to revolutionize patient care by enhancing diagnostic accuracy, improving treatment plans, and optimizing health-care workflows. However, achieving these benefits requires seamless collaboration between artificial intelligence developers and health-care professionals. This chapter examines the foundation of the existing gaps between these groups, explores critical knowledge, and proposes strategies to foster effective interdisciplinary partnerships. By addressing these challenges, artificial intelligence solutions can be aligned with clinical needs, ensuring they are both user-friendly and impactful in improving health-care outcomes.

Keywords

Collaboration · Clinical workflow · Interdisciplinary education · Communication barriers · Explainable artificial intelligence · Diagnostic accuracy · Ethical considerations

6.1 Foundation for the Gap Between Artificial Intelligence Developers and Health-Care Professionals

Applying artificial intelligence in health care presents transformative opportunities to enhance the quality, efficiency, and personalization of patient care, but its success hinges on effective collaboration between artificial intelligence developers and health-care professionals. The root of the existing gap between these two groups lies primarily in disparate educational backgrounds, limited opportunities for interdisciplinary communication, reliance on individual efforts for continuous learning, and the rapid evolution of digital health technology. These underlying challenges form

T. Hirosawa, *Artificial Intelligence in Medical Diagnostics*,
https://doi.org/10.1007/978-981-95-4338-0_6

the bottom layer of obstacles that hinder seamless integration and collaboration. Addressing these root issues is essential to maximize the collaborative potential of artificial intelligence and health care.

6.1.1 Education Backgrounds

Artificial intelligence developers typically have backgrounds in fields like computer science, engineering, or data science, focusing on technical competencies such as algorithm design, computational models, machine learning, and software development. These professionals prioritize algorithmic efficiency, accuracy, scalability, and technological innovation. In contrast, health-care professionals are educated within medical disciplines, emphasizing anatomy, pathology, clinical diagnosis, patient-centered care, and therapeutic practices. Their focus tends toward clinical effectiveness, patient safety, ethical considerations, and practical implementation within health systems.

This divergence in educational backgrounds leads to differing terms, values, and approaches. Artificial intelligence developers might prioritize technological feasibility and optimization, while health-care professionals emphasize clinical efficiency, patient safety, and ethical compliance. Such differences resonate with C. P. Snow's "Two Cultures" concepts, which describe the profound divide between scientific and literacy intellectuals, each largely unfamiliar with the other's foundational knowledge [1, 2]. Although the analogy is not perfect, the essence of Snow's framework describes the challenges inherent in merging artificial intelligence and medical disciplines. Bridging this gap demands deliberate educational interventions that foster mutual understanding and shared language.

6.1.2 Limited Opportunities for Interdisciplinary Updates

Traditional medical education mainly emphasizes clinical expertise and knowledge, with limited coverage of emerging technologies such as artificial intelligence or digital health tools. As a result, many health-care professionals enter practice without foundational knowledge in data science, computational methods, or digital infrastructure. This curricular gap leaves health-care professionals underprepared to engage with artificial intelligence technologies.

In addition, structured platforms for interdisciplinary learning—such as collaborative workshops or integrated technology modules in medical training—are scarce. Continuing medical education programs that address digital health remain underdeveloped, inconsistently implemented, and poorly incentivized. Without regular, institutionally supported opportunities for cross-disciplinary learning, the gap between artificial intelligence and clinical practice continues to grow, hampering effective collaboration [3].

6.1.3 Reliance on Individual Efforts

In the absence of systematic educational support, many health-care professionals must pursue artificial intelligence literacy independently. Overreliance on personal initiative leads to inequities in digital proficiency, as individuals face varying constraints related to time, access to resources, and interest in technology. Consequently, digital literacy levels across the health-care workforce are uneven. Digital literacy is detailed in Chap. 14.

Health-care professionals with prior technical experience or strong interest in digital tools may become informal mediators in artificial intelligence and health-care collaborations, while others remain disengaged. This uneven distribution of expertise impedes the broad adoption of artificial intelligence technologies and centralizes knowledge in a few individuals, limiting scalability and sustainability.

6.1.4 Rapid Evolution of Digital Health

The field of digital health, including artificial intelligence applications, is marked by constant and rapid innovation. New algorithms, platforms, and tools emerge regularly, driven by exponential growth in computational capacity, as exemplified by Moore's law. The law predicts that the number of transistors on a microchip doubles approximately every 2 years, thereby exponentially increasing computing power while reducing relative cost [4]. For instance, between 1979 and 2019, transistor counts in computer processors increased dramatically from 68×10^3 to 32×10^9, enabling the development of increasingly complex artificial intelligence models [5]. On the other hand, health-care professionals face substantial barriers in understanding and leveraging these continually emerging technological resources without structured training and supportive educational frameworks.

Amara's law further complicates this dynamic, suggesting that people tend to overestimate the short-term impact of new technologies while underestimating their long-term implications [6]. This can result in both inflated expectations and early disappointment, further complicating the integration of artificial intelligence into health care systems.

To bridge the divide between artificial intelligence developers and health-care professionals, strategic interventions are essential. These include embedding artificial intelligence education into medical training, promoting structured and recurring interdisciplinary collaboration, and fostering joint research and development initiatives. Building a shared terminology and aligning mutual objectives will create a foundation for meaningful collaboration. Ultimately, such efforts will enable both fields to advance in harmony, unlocking artificial intelligence's full potential to support compassionate, effective, and innovative health care. Beyond these structural challenges, health-care professionals also need a clear understanding of artificial intelligence itself—its scope, limitations, and ethical implications.

6.2 What Health-Care Professionals Should Know About Artificial Intelligence

For effective collaboration with artificial intelligence technologies, health-care professionals must develop a foundational understanding of artificial intelligence's capabilities, limitations, and evolving role within clinical practice. Key areas requiring particular attention include clearly defining what constitutes artificial intelligence, addressing the black box problem inherent in some artificial intelligence systems, and navigating associated ethical considerations.

6.2.1 Understanding What Constitutes Artificial Intelligence

Artificial intelligence in health care is frequently misunderstood as encompassing all computer-based solutions. Artificial intelligence specifically refers to advanced computational methods, including machine learning, deep learning, neural networks, and natural language processing. These sophisticated techniques enable computers to learn from large datasets, identify patterns, and make predictions or recommendations without explicit programming instructions.

However, it is crucial for health-care professionals to recognize that artificial intelligence is not always the most suitable approach for every clinical problem. In some cases, traditional rule-based systems, statistical modeling, or simple decision trees may provide more transparent, cost-effective, and equally reliable solutions. For instance, daily diagnostic decision-making typically benefits from simpler algorithms that offer clarity and easier interpretation compared to complex artificial intelligence models [7, 8].

The development and deployment of artificial intelligence in clinical settings is not purely a scientific endeavor but also an art form, resonating deeply with the nuanced nature of medicine itself. Selecting appropriate artificial intelligence models involves significant expertise and judgment—such as deciding whether a neural network is necessary, adjusting the number of layers within it, or choosing optimal hyperparameters to refine performance. This intricate interplay between structured scientific methodology and intuitive, creative decision-making characterizes the artistry inherent in artificial intelligence development.

Generative artificial intelligence platforms highlight the blend of technical precision and creative strategy involved in artificial intelligence applications. Developers must thoughtfully set and continually refine safety parameters to prevent misinformation or amplification of biases, reflecting a delicate balance between innovation and ethical responsibility. Effective use of generative artificial intelligence also demands skilled prompt engineering, where the clarity and precision of user input significantly influence the quality and appropriateness of outputs. Moreover, developers must fine-tune models by manipulating adjustable parameters: adjusting the system prompt, setting the "Top P" parameter to constrain token selection to a probabilistically diverse subset, and modifying the "temperature" value to control the degree of creativity and variability in the output. Such subtle calibrations can profoundly affect the model's interpretability and trustworthiness in a medical context, thereby demonstrating how nuanced design decisions, both ethical and aesthetic, ultimately shape clinical utility and patient safety [9].

6.2.2 "Black Box" Problem

A significant challenge in adopting artificial intelligence in health care is the "black box" problem, where the internal decision-making processes of complex artificial intelligence models remain difficult to interpret [10, 11]. This lack of transparency raises critical questions about reliability, accountability, and clinical trustworthiness. Health-care professionals must understand the implications of integrating systems whose outputs cannot be easily validated, particularly in complex scenarios such as diagnostic accuracy, treatment recommendations, or predicting patient outcomes.

For example, in radiology, deep learning models may identify subtle imaging features associated with lung cancer, yet fail to provide clear reasoning for why one image is classified as malignant while another is not [12, 13]. Health-care professionals are then left uncertain about whether the model is recognizing relevant pathological features or simply exploiting unrelated patterns in the data. Similarly, in cardiology, predictive algorithms have been developed to estimate a patient's risk of sudden cardiac arrest, but their decision-making criteria are often opaque, making it difficult for physicians to explain or justify recommendations to patients [14]. These situations highlight how lack of interpretability can hinder clinical adoption, reduce trust, and complicate shared decision-making.

Addressing the "black box" problem requires active advocacy by health-care professionals for more transparent, interpretable artificial intelligence. Explainable artificial intelligence technologies, which provide clear, understandable rationales for decisions, are becoming increasingly essential. By adopting explainable artificial intelligence approaches, health-care professionals can better evaluate artificial intelligence's reliability, communicate decisions clearly to patients, and maintain trust and accountability in clinical practice.

Beyond a lack of interpretability, the "black box" can also hide other dangers. Therefore, understanding the potential risks associated with artificial intelligence systems is essential. Hidden biases, additional risks, or unrecognized limitations may inadvertently lead to errors, negatively impacting patient safety. Professionals must remain alert, routinely evaluate artificial intelligence performance, and advocate for rigorous validation and continuous monitoring of deployed systems.

6.2.3 Ethical Considerations

Health-care professionals must navigate several complex ethical challenges when incorporating artificial intelligence into clinical settings. Foremost among these challenges is safeguarding patient privacy and data security. Establishing secure data infrastructures and adhering to stringent data governance standards can protect sensitive patient information.

Equally critical is addressing biases embedded within artificial intelligence systems. Biases can arise from limited, nonrepresentative training datasets and may lead to disparities in clinical outcomes, disproportionately affecting certain patient populations [15, 16]. To mitigate these risks, professionals should advocate for the development and utilization of diverse, representative datasets during the artificial intelligence training phase, actively working toward equitable and unbiased care.

Lastly, striking an appropriate balance between technological efficiency and human oversight is essential. Although artificial intelligence can dramatically enhance efficiency and accuracy, human judgment, empathy, and compassion must remain central to patient care. Maintaining this balance ensures that technological advancements enhance rather than diminish the human aspects of clinical interactions, reinforcing patient-centered care and preserving the fundamental ethical standards of health-care practice.

6.3 What Artificial Intelligence Developers Should Know About Health Care

Artificial intelligence developers must cultivate a comprehensive understanding of the distinct complexities within the health-care system and clinical workflows where their solutions will be implemented. This involves more than technical expertise. It necessitates awareness and appreciation of the foundational principles guiding health care, an in-depth understanding of clinical workflows, sensitivity toward user-centric design, awareness of interdisciplinary collaboration dynamics, and adherence to ethical and legal standards.

6.3.1 Understanding the Foundational Elements of Health Care

Health care operates upon core principles that include patient-centered care, evidence-based practice, and ethical decision-making. Patient-centered care emphasizes tailoring interventions to individual patient needs, preferences, and values, ensuring that clinical decisions support personalized outcomes. Developers must understand that effective artificial intelligence tools must enhance, not replace, health-care professionals' judgment and patient-health care professional relationships and should be designed to support and augment empathy-driven patient interactions.

Evidence-based practice ensures clinical decisions are grounded in scientifically validated literature, promoting safe and effective patient care. Artificial intelligence developers need to integrate evidence-based methodologies into artificial intelligence algorithms, ensuring recommendations are transparent, credible, and verifiable by health-care professionals [17].

Ethical decision-making is crucial, given the sensitive nature of health care. Artificial intelligence developers must design solutions that respect patient autonomy, privacy, confidentiality, and shared decision-making. Developers must proactively address ethical challenges that could arise from artificial intelligence applications, such as algorithmic biases or automated decision-making affecting patient outcomes.

6.3.2 Understanding the Clinical Workflow

Health-care workflows are dynamic and context-sensitive and vary considerably across different environments. Clinical settings like hospitals, outpatient clinics, nursing facilities, telemedicine platforms, and emergency departments each have unique operational frameworks. Specialties, including radiology, oncology, cardiology, and primary care, each exhibit distinct clinical pathways, documentation practices, and decision-making processes.

Geographical and seasonal contexts further influence workflow dynamics [18, 19]. In colder climates, seasonal influenza significantly affects primary care and emergency department workflows, causing predictable but intense periods of increased demand. Conversely, hot and humid regions susceptible to vector-borne diseases, like dengue fever outbreaks in tropical areas, require agile and responsive clinical protocols. Artificial intelligence developers must design adaptive solutions capable of accommodating such variability.

Rural and urban disparities further highlight workflow differences. Rural health care often relies extensively on telemedicine to bridge gaps created by limited access to specialists, whereas urban centers typically offer more immediate, face-to-face care. Solutions must therefore be contextually aware and adjustable to fit seamlessly within existing workflows without introducing additional complexity.

6.3.3 Importance of User-Centric Design

Artificial intelligence developers must prioritize user-centric design principles to ensure usability within high-pressure clinical environments. Health-care professionals require intuitive, efficient, and reliable tools that seamlessly integrate into their daily routines. Developers should engage health-care professionals actively and iteratively throughout design, testing, and deployment stages, incorporating their feedback to refine interfaces, workflows, and outputs. User-centric design also mandates that artificial intelligence-generated outputs are interpretable, actionable, and clinically relevant. Artificial intelligence tools must present insights in straightforward, accessible formats that health-care professionals can quickly assimilate and act upon, enhancing rather than complicating decision-making processes [20].

Beyond clinical professionals, patients themselves can also be users of artificial intelligence solutions, particularly in telemedical contexts. For example, remote monitoring platforms that incorporate artificial intelligence can provide patients with personalized alerts about abnormal vital signs, medication adherence reminders, or tailored self-care recommendations [21]. In such cases, design must account for patients' varying levels of digital literacy, health literacy, and accessibility needs. Interfaces should be simple, transparent, and supportive, helping patients feel empowered rather than overwhelmed by technology. By considering both health-care professional and patient perspectives, artificial intelligence developers can create solutions that strengthen the therapeutic alliance, improve adherence, and foster trust in digital health tools.

6.3.4 Collaborative Nature of Health Care

Health-care delivery relies on coordinated efforts across interdisciplinary teams, involving health-care professionals, nurses, technicians, therapists, and administrative staff. Artificial intelligence developers must recognize and support this collaboration through technologies that facilitate effective communication, seamless information exchange, and coordinated care planning.

Rather than promoting isolated use, artificial intelligence solutions should enhance team-based interactions by integrating with existing communication and collaboration systems. Developers should aim to foster transparency and coherence among team members, enabling shared understanding and collaborative decision-making.

6.3.5 Ethical and Legal Implications

Artificial intelligence solutions in health care must align strictly with established ethical standards and legal regulations. Developers need comprehensive knowledge of health information privacy laws such as the Health Insurance Portability and Accountability Act in the United States and the General Data Protection Regulation in Europe [22, 23]. Compliance involves protecting patient data, ensuring secure data handling practices, and maintaining rigorous confidentiality standards.

Furthermore, developers should actively address potential biases in artificial intelligence algorithms by utilizing diverse and representative datasets during model training to minimize inequities. Human oversight must be maintained, particularly in high-stakes decisions, to ensure accountability, transparency, and patient safety.

Overall, developers must proactively engage with complexity, ethics, workflows, and collaboration intrinsic to health care, fostering artificial intelligence solutions that are clinically relevant, ethically sound, and practically effective.

6.4 Bridging the Gap: Strategies for Collaboration

Effective collaboration between artificial intelligence developers and health-care professionals requires intentional efforts to bridge their differences. Strategies include interdisciplinary education and training, collaborative research and development, development of common standards, and incentivizing collaboration.

6.4.1 Interdisciplinary Education and Training

One of the most effective approaches involves interdisciplinary education and training. Health-care professionals should be provided with accessible resources, such as workshops, online courses, and certifications, that introduce artificial intelligence fundamentals tailored to the health-care context. These educational opportunities would enable health-care professionals to grasp the capabilities and limitations of artificial intelligence, fostering more informed usage of artificial intelligence tools [24]. Conversely, developers would benefit from shadowing health-care professionals and observing real-world medical workflows, helping them design artificial intelligence solutions that align closely with clinical realities.

Exploratory initiatives in this area include programs such as the Massachusetts Institute of Technology–Harvard Health Sciences and Technology Artificial Intelligence in Medicine curriculum, which has piloted courses combining medical case-based learning with machine learning methods [25]. Similarly, the University of Florida is infusing artificial intelligence across the curriculum and developing opportunities for student engagement within identified areas of artificial intelligence literacy regardless of student discipline [26]. This kind of broad-based integration demonstrates how interdisciplinary education can cultivate a culture of artificial intelligence fluency, preparing both health-care professionals and developers to collaborate more effectively.

6.4.2 Collaborative Research and Development

Collaborative research and development initiatives also play a pivotal role in bridging the gap. Joint projects that bring together health-care professionals, developers, and data scientists can lead to the creation of artificial intelligence tools that are not only technically robust but also clinically relevant. Co-creation processes, where health-care professionals actively participate in the design and testing phases, ensure that the tools are user-friendly and meet the practical needs of health-care providers.

A notable example of exploratory collaboration is the Stanford Center for Artificial Intelligence in Medicine and Imaging, which fosters collaboration among health care professionals, engineers, and researchers to explore novel artificial intelligence applications in radiology and imaging sciences [27]. The initiative demonstrates how collaborative environments can accelerate innovation while ensuring clinical applicability.

6.4.3 Development of Common Standards

The establishment of common standards is another essential strategy. By using simple language and clear concepts that avoid medical jargon and artificial intelligence-specific terminology, shared terminologies and frameworks can facilitate clearer communication between the two groups. This approach ensures that health-care professionals and artificial intelligence developers can work together without misinterpretation or confusion caused by specialized vocabulary. Furthermore, developing standardized protocols for artificial intelligence implementation in health care can ensure consistency, reliability, and interoperability across various systems and institutions, creating a shared understanding that bridges their differing professional languages. Early exploratory work toward such standards includes the World Health Organization's guidance on ethics and governance of artificial intelligence in health, which proposed frameworks for responsible artificial intelligence deployment [28].

6.4.4 Incentivizing Collaboration

Incentivizing collaboration is crucial for sustaining these efforts. Providing funding and institutional support for interdisciplinary projects encourages innovative solutions. Recognizing and rewarding teams that successfully integrate artificial intelligence into clinical practice serves as an additional motivation, promoting a culture of collaboration and shared success.

6.4.5 Intersectional Terms in Artificial Intelligence and Medicine

To bridge the gap between artificial intelligence developers and health-care professionals, it is essential to recognize the varying interpretations of intersectional terms. These terms, whose meanings shift depending on the context, can lead to misunderstanding unless clearly defined. A detailed overview of representative intersectional terms is provided in Table 6.1.

In radiology, the term "AI" occasionally refers to autopsy imaging, involving advanced computational tools to enhance postmortem radiological analysis [29]. In general technology and computer science, "AI" or artificial intelligence refers to systems capable of sophisticated tasks like predictive analytics, decision support, and autonomous problem-solving.

"Hallucination" traditionally describes sensory perceptions that occur without external stimuli, commonly associated with psychiatric or neurological conditions, such as schizophrenia [30]. In the context of large language models, "hallucination" refers to the generation of outputs that are incorrect, or illogical [31]. This occurs because large language models generate outputs based on probabilistic patterns derived from previously learned data, without intrinsic comprehension of real-world contexts. Conversely, health-care professionals rely fundamentally on clinical knowledge, physiological insights, and anatomical understanding for accurate diagnostics. Large language models, lacking this intrinsic understanding, may produce misleading outputs. Although iterative models have improved in accuracy and decreased "hallucinations" [32], this limitation highlights the necessity of continual human review, especially when artificial intelligence is applied in sensitive domains like health care.

Table 6.1 Representative intersectional terms in artificial intelligence and medicine

Term	Meaning in medicine	Meaning in artificial intelligence
AI	In a radiology context, "AI" occasionally refers to autopsy imaging, where advanced computational tools are employed to enhance and streamline postmortem radiological analysis	In the broader domain of technology, "AI," artificial intelligence, encapsulates the development of systems capable of tasks like predictive modeling and decision support
Hallucination	Sensory perception in the absence of external stimulus, often associated with neurological or psychiatric conditions (e.g., symptoms of schizophrenia)	Generating factually incorrect, nonsensical, or ungrounded outputs, especially in large language models
Sensitivity	Ability of a test to correctly identify individuals *with* a disease (true positive rate)	True positive rate of a classification model; the proportion of actual positives correctly identified
Specificity	Ability of a test to correctly identify individuals *without* a disease (true negative rate)	True negative rate of a classification model; the proportion of actual negatives correctly identified
Bias	Systematic errors in a study or a prejudice that can lead to unfair outcomes	Systemic flaws in data (e.g., unrepresentative datasets) or algorithms that result in unfair or discriminatory outcomes
Overfitting	Relying too heavily on specific tests/ symptoms, leading to incomplete diagnosis	Model learns training data too well (including noise), performing poorly on new data; fails to generalize
Generalization	Applying study findings to a broader population	Ability of a trained model to perform well on new, unseen data
Validation	Confirming accuracy and reliability of a test, treatment, or research finding	Evaluating a trained model's performance on a separate dataset, validation set, to assess generalization and avoid overfitting
Noise	Unwanted or irrelevant information interfering with a signal (e.g., artifacts on an electrocardiography)	Irrelevant or inconsistent data points that impair model training and performance
Confidence	A degree of certainty (e.g., in a diagnosis)	A numerical score indicating the probability assigned by the model to a certain prediction
Black box	A complex process or mechanism that is not fully understood	Models (especially deep learning) whose internal workings are difficult to interpret or understand
Feedback loop	Physiological processes where output influences input, creating a cycle (e.g., blood glucose regulation). In medical education: A process where learners receive information on their performance, which they can use to improve future performance	Processes where outputs of an AI system are used to improve its performance over time, particularly in adapting to new data and clinical scenarios in medicine

(continued)

Table 6.1 (continued)

Term	Meaning in medicine	Meaning in artificial intelligence
Temperature	Commonly, body temperature, one of vital signs	Factor controlled the randomness and creativity of the model's output, with lower settings yielding more predictable results and higher settings increasing variability (detailed in Chap. 8)
Vision	Physiological and neurological process of sight to perceive the world through the eyes and interpret the information received	Enabling computers to interpret images and videos
Dropout	Participants who withdraw from a study before its completion in clinical research	A regularization technique to deactivate a proportion of nodes in a layer within training iteration of neural network

"Sensitivity" in clinical medicine denotes a diagnostic test's ability to correctly identify patients who truly have the disease, thus representing the true positive rate [33]. In artificial intelligence classification, sensitivity similarly refers to the true positive rate, measuring the model's effectiveness in identifying positive instances accurately, as further discussed in Chap. 1.

"Specificity" signifies the ability of a test to correctly identify individuals without a disease, which is the true negative rate [33]. Similarly, in artificial intelligence, "specificity" represents the true negative rate of a classification model, indicating the proportion of actual negatives correctly identified, detailed in Chap. 1.

In clinical contexts, "bias" often manifests as cognitive bias—systematic errors in reasoning or decision-making processes that can negatively affect diagnostic accuracy and patient outcomes. Examples include confirmation bias, where health-care professionals selectively interpret symptoms to confirm a preconceived diagnosis, potentially leading to misdiagnosis. In artificial intelligence, "bias" refers to systemic discrepancies embedded in data or algorithmic designs, inadvertently producing discriminatory or unfair outcomes. Artificial intelligence "bias" may originate from unrepresentative datasets or algorithmic flaws, disproportionately affecting minority or underrepresented groups. Thus, "bias" in artificial intelligence necessitates rigorous mitigation through balanced datasets, fairness-aware algorithms, and continuous oversight, as thoroughly discussed in Chap. 1.

"Overfitting" within clinical medicine pertains to excessive reliance on specific tests or symptoms, possibly overlooking broader clinical context and resulting in inaccurate diagnoses. In artificial intelligence, overfitting refers to a model's excessive memorization of the training dataset, including irrelevant details or noise, impairing performance on new or unseen data [34].

"Generalization" in clinical research describes the applicability of findings to broader patient populations. Similarly, artificial intelligence generalization reflects the capability of models to maintain performance consistency across previously unseen data.

"Validation" signifies the confirmation of accuracy and reliability in clinical diagnostics or treatments. In the context of artificial intelligence, "validation" involves assessing a model's effectiveness using separate "validation" datasets, ensuring robust performance and preventing overfitting.

"Noise" refers to unwanted or irrelevant information interfering with a signal, such as artifacts on an electrocardiography. In diagnostic context, "noise," often referred to as a "red herring," can lead health-care professionals astray by presenting misleading information that draws attention away from the actual diagnosis [35]. For example, in a complex diagnostic case involving chest pain, a health-care professional might focus on gastrointestinal symptoms and pursue a diagnosis of gastroesophageal reflux disease, while the true cause could be a cardiac event. Similarly, in artificial intelligence, "noise" represents errors, inconsistencies, or irrelevant data points in a dataset that can negatively impact model training and performance.

"Confidence" indicates a degree of certainty, such as in a diagnosis. In artificial intelligence, "Confidence" is a numerical score indicating the probability assigned by the model to a certain prediction.

A "black box" is a complex process or mechanism that is not fully understood. In artificial intelligence, "black box" refers to models, especially in deep learning, whose internal workings are difficult to interpret or understand.

"Feedback loop" describes physiological processes where output influences subsequent activity. In artificial intelligence, a "feedback loop" refers to a process where outputs of an artificial intelligence system influence subsequent inputs or model adjustments.

"Temperature," in a physiological context, represents the commonly measured body temperature, one of the vital signs. In the realm of artificial intelligence, particularly in the context of language models, "temperature" is a factor that controls the randomness and creativity of the model's output, with lower settings yielding more predictable results and higher settings increasing variability [36], as detailed in Chap. 8.

"Vision" describes the physiological and neurological process of sight, perceiving the world through the eyes and interpreting the information received. In artificial intelligence, "vision" or computer vision is a field focused on enabling computers to interpret images and videos.

In clinical research, "dropout" refers to participants who withdraw from a study before its completion. In the context of artificial intelligence, "dropout" is a regularization technique to deactivate a proportion of nodes in a layer during each training iteration of a neural network, preventing overfitting and improving model generalization.

In summary, bridging the gap between artificial intelligence developers and health-care professionals is essential for unlocking the full potential of artificial intelligence in health care. By fostering mutual understanding and collaboration, these groups can create innovative, effective, and ethical solutions that improve patient care and advance medical science. This chapter lays the foundation for exploring the practical applications of artificial intelligence in health care, emphasizing the importance of teamwork and shared knowledge in shaping the future of medicine.

References

1. Snow CP. Two cultures. Science (New York, NY). 1959;130(3373):419.
2. Jacobs SCP. Snow's the two cultures: Michael Polanyi's response and context. Bull Sci Technol Soc. 2011;31(3):172–8.
3. Tolsgaard MG, Boscardin CK, Park YS, Cuddy MM, Sebok-Syer SS. The role of data science and machine learning in Health Professions Education: practical applications, theoretical contributions, and epistemic beliefs. Adv Health Sci Educ. 2020;25(5):1057–86.
4. Moore GE. Cramming more components onto integrated circuits. Electronics. 1965;38:114–7.
5. Delipetrev B, Tsinaraki, C. and Kostic, U. Historical evolution of artificial intelligence. Luxembourg: Publications Office of the European Union; 2020.
6. Amara R. Some observations on the interaction of technology and society. Futures. 1975;7(6):515–7.
7. Wang H, Fu T, Du Y, Gao W, Huang K, Liu Z, et al. Scientific discovery in the age of artificial intelligence. Nature. 2023;620(7972):47–60.
8. Messeri L, Crockett M. Artificial intelligence and illusions of understanding in scientific research. Nature. 2024;627(8002):49–58.
9. Abiodun OI, Jantan A, Omolara AE, Dada KV, Mohamed NA, Arshad H. State-of-the-art in artificial neural network applications: a survey. Heliyon. 2018;4(11):e00938.
10. Ford RA, Price W, Nicholson I. Privacy and accountability in black-box medicine. Mich Telecommun Tech L Rev. 2016;23:1.
11. Price W, Nicholson I. Regulating black-box medicine. Mich L Rev. 2017;116:421.
12. Raghu VK, Walia AS, Zinzuwadia AN, Goiffon RJ, Shepard J-AO, Aerts HJWL, et al. Validation of a deep learning–based model to predict lung cancer risk using chest radiographs and electronic medical record data. JAMA Netw Open. 2022;5(12):e2248793-e.
13. Zhang Q-s, Zhu S-c. Visual interpretability for deep learning: a survey. Front Inf Technol Electron Eng. 2018;19(1):27–39.
14. Petch J, Di S, Nelson W. Opening the black box: the promise and limitations of explainable machine learning in cardiology. Can J Cardiol. 2022;38(2):204–13.
15. Panch T, Mattie H, Atun R. Artificial intelligence and algorithmic bias: implications for health systems. J Glob Health. 2019;9(2):010318.
16. Zhou N, Zhang Z, Nair VN, Singhal H, Chen J. Bias, fairness and accountability with artificial intelligence and machine learning algorithms. Int Stat Rev. 2022;90(3):468–80.
17. Patrick TB, Demiris G, Folk LC, Moxley DE, Mitchell JA, Tao D. Evidence-based retrieval in evidence-based medicine. J Med Libr Assoc. 2004;92(2):196–9.
18. Valenčius CB. Histories of medical geography. Med Hist. 2000;44(S20):3–28.
19. Stewart S, Keates AK, Redfern A, McMurray JJ. Seasonal variations in cardiovascular disease. Nat Rev Cardiol. 2017;14(11):654–64.
20. Rožanec JM, Inna N, Patrik Z, Klemen K, Hooman TG, Sungho S, et al. Human-centric artificial intelligence architecture for Industry 5.0 applications. Int J Prod Res. 2023;61(20):6847–72.
21. Lu T, Lin Q, Yu B, Hu J. A systematic review of strategies in digital technologies for motivating adherence to chronic illness self-care. NPJ Health Syst. 2025;2(1):13.
22. Act A. Health insurance portability and accountability act of 1996. Public Law. 1996;104:191.
23. Forcier MB, Gallois H, Mullan S, Joly Y. Integrating artificial intelligence into health care through data access: can the GDPR act as a beacon for policymakers? J Law Biosci. 2019;6(1):317–35.
24. Baturalp TB, Bozkurt S, Baldock C. The future of biomedical engineering education is transdisciplinary. Phys Eng Sci Med. 2024:1–4.

25. Burns-Hernandez LU, Greenberg JE. Harvard-MIT division of health sciences and technology. IEEE Pulse. 2011;2(4):68–9.
26. Southworth J, Migliaccio K, Glover J, Glover JN, Reed D, McCarty C, et al. Developing a model for AI Across the curriculum: transforming the higher education landscape via innovation in AI literacy. Comput Educ Artif Intell. 2023;4:100127.
27. Langlotz CP, Kim J, Shah N, Lungren MP, Larson DB, Datta S, et al. Developing a research center for artificial intelligence in medicine. Mayo Clin Proc Digit Health. 2024;2(4):677–86.
28. WHO. Ethics and governance of artificial intelligence for health: WHO guidance. 2021.
29. Bolliger SA, Thali MJ, Ross S, Buck U, Naether S, Vock P. Virtual autopsy using imaging: bridging radiologic and forensic sciences. A review of the Virtopsy and similar projects. Eur Radiol. 2008;18:273–82.
30. Waters F, Fernyhough C. Hallucinations: a systematic review of points of similarity and difference across diagnostic classes. Schizophr Bull. 2017;43(1):32–43.
31. Huang L, Yu W, Ma W, Zhong W, Feng Z, Wang H, et al. A survey on hallucination in large language models: principles, taxonomy, challenges, and open questions. ACM Trans Inf Syst. 2024;43:1–55.
32. OpenAI. GPT-4 technical report. arXiv e-prints. 2023:arXiv:2303.08774.
33. Sackett DL. The rational clinical examination. A primer on the precision and accuracy of the clinical examination. JAMA. 1992;267(19):2638–44.
34. Santos CFGD, Papa JP. Avoiding overfitting: a survey on regularization methods for convolutional neural networks. ACM Comput Surv. 2022;54(10s):213.
35. Zweifel P. The 'red herring' hypothesis: some theory and new evidence. Healthcare (Basel). 2022;10(2):211.
36. Choi J, Lee B. Accelerating materials language processing with large language models. Commun Mater. 2024;5(1):13.

7 Useful Concept of AI in Diagnostics

Abstract

Artificial intelligence is revolutionizing the medical field, especially in diagnostics. It bridges complex technical concepts and clinical applications, allowing health-care professionals to leverage its capabilities effectively. A critical appraisal for artificial intelligence outputs is discussed, emphasizing the importance of evaluating artificial intelligence-generated data with the same rigor applied to traditional research methodologies. Additionally, this chapter provides an in-depth exploration of key artificial intelligence concepts. Furthermore, this chapter provides the challenges of adopting these concepts in clinically relevant contexts.

Keywords

Backpropagation · Quantification · Overfitting · Ensemble · Transfer learning · Dropout · Reversed prompt engineering

7.1 Overview of Useful AI Concepts

While health-care professionals will not be directly implementing backpropagation or quantification like artificial intelligence developers, understanding these concepts can help them better utilize and evaluate artificial intelligence tools. Certain concepts would be particularly valuable for health-care professionals to adopt due to their clinical relevance.

In essence, these concepts highlight the following:

- Artificial intelligence learns from data, just like health-care professionals learn from experience. The quality and diversity of that data are important.
- Artificial intelligence relies on the quantity, quality, and diversity of the input data. The more objective, standardized, and representative the clinical observations are, the better an artificial intelligence can potentially assist you.

T. Hirosawa, *Artificial Intelligence in Medical Diagnostics*,
https://doi.org/10.1007/978-981-95-4338-0_7

- Artificial intelligence models can be overconfident or biased. Critical evaluation and understanding of a model's limitations, such as critical appraisal, are crucial.
- Combining different perspectives, whether from multiple artificial intelligence models or multiple health-care professionals, often leads to better outcomes.

In the following sections, a critical appraisal for artificial intelligence outputs is discussed, emphasizing the importance of evaluating artificial intelligence-generated data with the same rigor applied to traditional research methodologies. Following this, several artificial intelligence-related terms are introduced, then clinical adoption for these concepts is explored.

7.2 Critical Appraisal of Artificial Intelligence Outputs

The process of integrating artificial intelligence also demands a critical appraisal mindset akin to evaluating traditional research articles [1]. In appraising research articles, health-care professionals examine the study's methodology, ensuring the research design is robust and minimizes biases. This includes evaluating the selection of participants, the appropriateness of interventions, the clarity in data collection procedures, and the robustness of statistical analysis. They critically assess the validity of the findings by questioning whether the data supports the conclusions drawn and whether the interpretations align with the study objectives. Additionally, the reproducibility of results is pivotal, requiring that methodologies be transparent enough to allow independent replication. Transparency is critical, with detailed descriptions of all steps in the research process ensuring credibility and applicability to real-world scenarios.

Similarly, artificial intelligence outputs require rigorous evaluation. This involves scrutinizing the quality and representativeness of data used to train the artificial intelligence models. It is essential to ensure this data aligns with diverse and clinically relevant populations. While trained data for artificial intelligence models is often not publicly available, the origin and preprocessing must be transparent to evaluate potential biases or limitations accurately. Medical textbooks provide foundational, peer-reviewed benchmarks for accuracy, while secondary resources like BMJ Best Practice, UpToDate®, and DynaMed® offer evidence-based summaries contextualizing artificial intelligence outputs within current clinical practices [2]. Original research articles further inform critical appraisal by introducing specific, cutting-edge insights and methodologies that can validate artificial intelligence performance.

In addition to reviewing the source data, the performance of the artificial intelligence model must be evaluated using metrics such as accuracy, precision, recall, and robustness across diverse datasets. Transparency in artificial intelligence demands clear documentation of the algorithms, the logic of decision-making processes, and a detailed understanding of model limitations. Validation is another cornerstone of critical appraisal, requiring external and independent validation using new datasets. This ensures artificial intelligence delivers consistent results, mirroring the validation requirements in traditional research through reproducibility and reliability testing.

Table 7.1 Comparing critical appraisal of traditional research medical articles and artificial intelligence (AI) outputs in medical context

Feature	Traditional research articles	AI outputs
Methodology	Robust research design Minimize biases Appropriate participant selection, interventions, data collection, and statistical analysis	Scrutinize data quality and representativeness Ensure data aligns with diverse and clinically relevant populations
Data source	Original research data collected during the study	Training data, often not publicly available Origin and preprocessing of training data must be transparent
Evaluation	Validity of findings, data supports conclusions Interpretations align with study objectives	Performance metrics, including accuracy, precision, recall, robustness Evaluate across diverse datasets
Transparency	Detailed descriptions of all research steps Methodologies transparent enough for independent replication	Clear documentation of algorithms and decision-making logic Understanding of model limitations Origin and preprocessing of training data should be available and transparent
Validation	Reproducibility of results Independent replication	External and independent validation using new datasets Consistent results, reproducibility and reliability
Resources	Primary sources such as research articles Secondary sources including clinical reference tools, reviews, and guidelines	Foundational: Medical textbooks Secondary: Evidence-based summaries Original research articles
Goal	Ensure credibility and applicability to real-world scenarios Improve patient care	Enhance trust in AI systems Ensure ethical responsibility and clinical applicability Improve patient care

A structured appraisal process that draws on trusted resources—from textbooks and secondary sources to original research—ensures the evaluation of artificial intelligence-generated outputs is as rigorous and thorough as the appraisal of medical research articles. Such diligence not only enhances trust in artificial intelligence systems but also ensures they are ethically responsible, clinically applicable, and aligned with the overarching goals of improving patient care. Comparing critical appraisal of traditional medical articles and artificial intelligence outputs in medical context is summarized in Table 7.1.

7.3 Backpropagation

In the following sections, several artificial intelligence-related terms are introduced; then clinical adoption for these concepts is explored [3].

7.3.1 Technical Meaning for Backpropagation

Backpropagation is the core algorithm behind how many artificial intelligence models, especially neural networks, "learn." It involves calculating the error between the model's prediction and the actual outcome; then adjusting the model's internal parameters, especially weights, to minimize this error; and propagating the corrections backward through the neural network [4]. Weights represent the strength of connection between different neurons in the neural network. A weight might be increased if it was too low and contributed to a wrong prediction or decreased if it was too high.

7.3.2 Clinical Adoption for Backpropagation

Conceptually, backpropagation can be thought of as a process of trial, error, and refinement. Artificial intelligence makes a guess, evaluates its error, and adjusts its approach for the next time. This iterative process mirrors a health-care professional's reflective practice: reviewing unexpected outcomes, analyzing causes, and improving future clinical practice.

When using artificial intelligence, remember that its prediction is based on prior data and might not apply perfectly to every patient. By understanding backpropagation, health-care professionals can better appreciate how artificial intelligence improves over time with more data.

7.4 Quantification

7.4.1 Technical Meaning for Quantification

Quantification is the process of representing information numerically. In artificial intelligence, this is crucial because models work with numbers [5]. It can involve assigning numerical scores to symptoms, measuring physiological parameters, or converting text or images into numerical representations.

7.4.2 Clinical Adoption for Quantification

Quantification is about finding ways to objectively measure aspects of a patient's condition or a clinical scenario so that artificial intelligence can process and analyze it. Health-care professionals should employ standard scales and measurements whenever possible, as these make assessments more objective and easier for artificial intelligence to interpret. For instance, a numeric rating scale ranging from 1 to 10 can be used to quantify symptoms, with 1 representing minimal severity and 10 indicating extreme severity [6]. Additionally, qualitative observations such as verbal rating scale, such as none, mild, moderate, and severe, can be translated into a numerical scale [7]. These quantifications are foundational for clinical prediction rules and improving diagnostic accuracy.

7.5 Avoid Overfitting

7.5.1 Technical Meaning for Overfitting

Overfitting occurs when an artificial intelligence model captures not only the true underlying pattern in the training data but also the noise and anomalies that are not representative of broader trends. As a result, the model becomes highly specialized in training data and loses its ability to generalize to new, unseen data. This leads to a decline in predictive accuracy when the model is applied outside its training environment [8]. For instance, when an artificial intelligence model was trained only on images of skin lesions from patients with certain skin types, the model might perform poorly when diagnosing skin cancer in patients with other skin types [9]. The model would have overfitted to the specific visual characteristics present in the limited dataset and failed to learn the broader, more generalizable features of skin lesions across diverse populations. This illustrates the importance of using balanced, representative datasets during training to ensure that artificial intelligence models can perform reliably across varied clinical contexts.

7.5.2 Clinical Adoption for Overfitting

In the clinical context, health-care professionals are trained in diverse environments, such as hospitals, clinics, rural health institutions, home visit medical treatment, and sometimes telemedical settings. This varied exposure ensures they acquire a broad understanding and adaptability to different situations. Similarly, health-care professionals should train artificial intelligence systems with diverse datasets to expose models to a variety of patient populations, helping them learn generalizable patterns. Additionally, they must remain aware of the limitations inherent in artificial intelligence models, critically evaluating their performance to ensure reliable application across different clinical scenarios.

7.6 Ensemble

7.6.1 Technical Meaning for Ensemble

Ensemble methods combine multiple artificial intelligence models to make a single prediction. The idea is that the collective wisdom of the "ensemble" is often more accurate and robust than any individual model. There are several ensemble techniques, but majority voting is the simplest, where multiple models predict an outcome, and the most frequent prediction is chosen as the result. Through these techniques, model performance is improved by reducing biases and increasing overall accuracy. Currently, deep learning architectures are demonstrating superior performance compared to traditional models. Ensemble learning combines the advantages of both deep learning models and ensemble techniques, leading to improved generalization performance. These models are categorized into approaches such as bagging, boosting, stacking, and negative correlation-based ensembles [10].

7.6.2 Clinical Adoption for Ensemble

Collective diagnosis plays a crucial role in medical decision-making, where multiple experts contribute their knowledge to refine conclusions [11]. Several studies have shown that collective diagnosis leads to improved outcomes compared to individual diagnosis, as it incorporates diverse perspectives and expertise, reducing errors and enhancing decision-making accuracy [12, 13]. Ensemble learning in artificial intelligence mirrors this approach by integrating multiple models to improve accuracy and reliability. Each model or expert may have unique strengths, and combining their output results in a more informed and balanced decision. In clinical settings, multidisciplinary collaborations, such as tumor boards and multidisciplinary conferences, enable specialists from different fields to provide diverse insights and collectively assess complex cases [14, 15]. Similarly, artificial intelligence-driven ensemble methods enhance diagnostic precision by aggregating predictions from different models, reducing bias, and increasing generalization performance. This collaborative approach, whether among health-care professionals or artificial intelligence systems, strengthens diagnostic accuracy and fosters better patient outcomes.

7.7 Transfer Learning

7.7.1 Technical Meaning for Transfer Learning

Transfer learning is a technique where a model trained on one task is adapted to a different but related task [16–18]. Instead of training a new model from scratch, you can leverage the knowledge gained from the previous task, as shown in Fig. 7.1. For example, a model trained to detect diabetic retinopathy (damage to blood vessels in the eye) could be fine-tuned to detect other retinal diseases [19].

7.7.2 Clinical Adoption for Transfer Learning

As introduced in Sect. 7.2, critical appraisal for research is also useful for evaluating artificial intelligence outputs. Just as health-care professionals meticulously assess research methodologies, data validity, and study reproducibility, they must

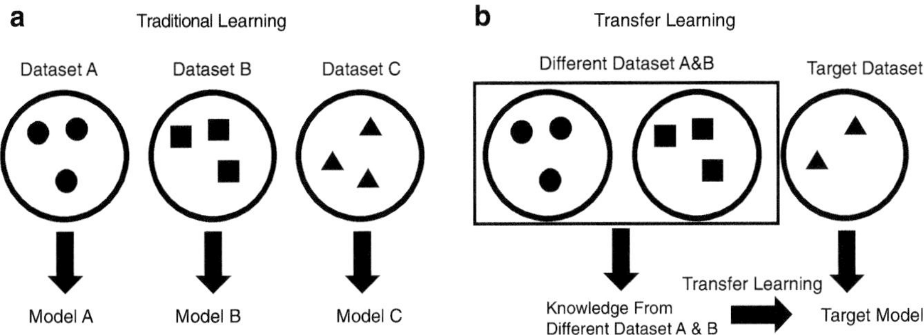

Fig. 7.1 Comparing the learning process in traditional learning versus transfer learning

apply the same level of scrutiny to outputs from artificial intelligence, especially in outputs related to medical diagnostics. By leveraging structured evaluation frameworks, health-care professionals can critically appraise artificial intelligence-generated recommendations, ensuring their reliability and clinical applicability.

For instance, outside of medicine, business strategies that emphasize leadership, process optimization, data-driven analysis, structured problem-solving, and risk assessment provide valuable frameworks that health-care professionals can integrate into medical reasoning [20, 21].

Similarly, engineering methodologies, particularly in the field of biomedical engineering, offer structured approaches for problem-solving and innovation that can be applied in medical contexts [22]. The collaboration between engineering and medicine fosters advancements in artificial intelligence-driven diagnostics, as engineers develop models optimized for medical applications while health-care professionals ensure their relevance and safety in patient care. By bridging these disciplines, health-care professionals can refine diagnostic processes, enhance predictive modeling, and improve overall treatment strategies through interdisciplinary collaboration [23, 24].

However, it is crucial to be cautious about overextending transfer learning methodologies from other fields and to consider domain-specific context [25]. While insights from other industries can be valuable, health-care decisions must align with ethical standards, patient background, and clinical nuances. Transfer learning should be adapted carefully to maintain clinical relevance and applicability. For instance, while cost-effectiveness is a valuable principle in medicine, excessively prioritizing it could lead to ethical concerns [26]. Similarly, a quantified approach to evaluating research performance could contribute to academic capitalism, where research value is determined primarily by numerical indicators rather than holistic clinical and social impact [27].

By leveraging methodologies from diverse fields, health-care professionals can refine their diagnostic accuracy and treatment strategies, improving patient outcomes through interdisciplinary approaches. The importance of interdisciplinary approaches is also discussed in Chap. 13.

7.8 Dropout

7.8.1 Technical Meaning for Dropout

Dropout is a regularization technique used during the training of neural networks. It involves randomly ignoring, "dropping out," a proportion of nodes and their connections during each training iteration. This prevents the network from relying too heavily on any specific neuron or feature, forcing it to learn more robust and generalizable representations. The term "dropout" is used in clinical research context and artificial intelligence context, detailed in Chap. 6.

7.8.2 Clinical Adoption for Dropout

Health-care professionals often "dropout" less relevant or inactive problems from the problem list to focus on the most pertinent issues for differential diagnosis. For example, in a complex case with multiple comorbidities, a health-care professional might initially list all problems (e.g., hypertension, diabetes mellitus, history of stroke, recent cough). However, to diagnose the cause of the cough, they might "drop out" the chronic conditions (hypertension, diabetes, stroke history) as less relevant to the acute issue, focusing instead on potential respiratory causes. This is analogous to a health-care professional temporarily "dropping out" less relevant data points to avoid being distracted from the core diagnostic problem. Experienced health-care professionals often unintentionally modify their problem lists depending on the diagnostic yield, adjusting their focus as new clinical information emerges. When dealing with a complex case, actively consider which problems are most relevant to the current presentation and temporarily "dropout" the less important ones to narrow your focus. Beyond model optimization techniques such as dropout, artificial intelligence also contributes directly to clinical image interpretation, for example, in identifying lesions of interest.

7.9 Lesion of Interest

7.9.1 Technical Meaning for Lesion of Interest

Within artificial intelligence-driven medical diagnostics, the term "lesion of interest" denotes specific regions within medical images that warrant closer clinical scrutiny due to their potential pathological significance. Advanced computer vision algorithms, including convolutional neural networks, deep learning-based segmentation methods, and anomaly detection techniques, are employed to pinpoint these lesions accurately and reliably across various imaging modalities such as X-rays, magnetic resonance imaging, computed tomography scans, ultrasound, and positron emission tomography [28].

These sophisticated artificial intelligence methods perform critical tasks. Image segmentation techniques differentiate lesions from normal tissue by delineating clear boundaries and providing volumetric measurements. Object detection algorithms identify and localize lesions in imaging scans, facilitating prompt and accurate assessment by health-care professionals. Additionally, anomaly detection approaches highlight deviations from normal anatomical patterns to flag potential abnormalities that might otherwise go unnoticed.

Integrating artificial intelligence-based lesion identification systems into clinical practice significantly enhances diagnostic precision. Such integration minimizes human error, reduces false negatives, and streamlines clinical workflows. By automatically identifying and annotating lesions of interest, artificial intelligence systems effectively support radiologists and health-care professionals, allowing them to concentrate their expertise on interpretation, diagnosis, and patient care strategies rather than exhaustive image evaluation.

7.9.2 Clinical Adoption for Lesion of Interest

Clinically, a "lesion of interest" is regarded as a targeted area of abnormal tissue or structure discovered through imaging modalities or clinical examinations, meriting further investigation due to its diagnostic or prognostic significance. Health-care professionals typically adopt individualized frameworks to identify and analyze "lesions of interest," often emphasizing criteria specific to their respective specialties. For instance, when evaluating feverish patients, health-care professionals may initially focus their framework on identifying bacterial infection sources through careful medical interviews and systematic physical examinations [29]. This focused approach, shaped by their clinical training and experience, helps guide diagnostic priorities and interpretations. Recognizing and understanding these individualized frameworks is crucial, as they influence how health-care professionals identify and interpret lesions or abnormalities in various clinical contexts.

Understanding these varied frameworks within clinical settings is essential, as clarity regarding each professional's perspective can significantly enhance interdisciplinary collaboration and improve diagnostic outcomes. Particularly in complex cases, health-care professionals may find it beneficial to broaden their scope of the "lesion of interest" beyond their initial diagnostic framework, considering alternative interpretations to uncover underlying causes that might not have been initially evident. For example, experienced health-care professionals managing a case of undiagnosed abdominal pain may begin by evaluating intra-abdominal structures. However, when initial imaging proves inconclusive, these professionals often extend their diagnostic framework beyond the abdomen. They may consider extra-abdominal or systemic causes such as pain from lower lobe pneumonia, diabetic ketoacidosis, porphyria, or anterior cutaneous nerve entrapment syndrome [30–32]. This flexible and integrative approach helps ensure comprehensive evaluation, accurate diagnosis, and effective patient management.

7.10 Reversed Prompt Engineering

7.10.1 Technical Meaning for Reversed Prompt Engineering

Reversed prompt engineering refers to the process of inferring or reconstructing the inputs or underlying logic that lead an artificial intelligence model to produce a particular output [33]. It is a reflective technique, allowing users to understand the internal mechanisms and decision pathways of complex artificial intelligence systems, particularly large language models. This approach enhances interpretability and transparency, offering insight into model behavior and helping to ensure outputs align with intended clinical objectives.

7.10.2 Clinical Adoption for Reversed Prompt Engineering

In clinical practice, reversed prompt engineering can be paralleled to a health-care professional's process of tracing back through diagnostic reasoning. For instance, when presented with a complex diagnosis, experienced health-care professionals may retrospectively analyze the patient's symptoms, history, and test results to understand how they arrived at their conclusion. This reflective approach is a fundamental part of clinical reasoning, fostering continuous learning and refinement of diagnostic skills [34–36]. Similarly, understanding artificial intelligence outputs by backtracking through the inputs and model logic ensures that predictions are grounded in clinically relevant data. Engaging in reflective practice while evaluating artificial intelligence not only enhances trust but also supports ethical accountability and facilitates the seamless integration of artificial intelligence into evidence-based clinical workflows. Prompt engineering is discussed in Sect. 8.3.4.

In conclusion, this chapter highlights the pivotal role of artificial intelligence in advancing medical diagnostics. From understanding key concepts like backpropagation and quantification to avoiding pitfalls such as overfitting, health-care professionals are better equipped to evaluate and utilize artificial intelligence tools. Techniques like ensemble methods and transfer learning demonstrate the adaptability and collaborative potential of artificial intelligence, while computer vision exemplifies its transformative impact in fields such as radiology and dermatology. To ensure these advancements translate into meaningful clinical outcomes, health-care professionals should harness the wisdom of the "ensemble" when integrating these technologies, critically evaluating their limitations, and fostering a synergy between artificial intelligence and traditional medical expertise.

References

1. Katrak P, Bialocerkowski AE, Massy-Westropp N, Kumar VSS, Grimmer KA. A systematic review of the content of critical appraisal tools. BMC Med Res Methodol. 2004;4(1):22.

2. Kwag KH, González-Lorenzo M, Banzi R, Bonovas S, Moja L. Providing doctors with high-quality information: an updated evaluation of web-based point-of-care information summaries. J Med Internet Res. 2016;18(1):e15.
3. Hirosawa T, Suzuki T, Shiraishi T, Hayashi A, Fujii Y, Harada T, et al. Adapting artificial intelligence concepts to enhance clinical decision-making: a hybrid intelligence framework. Int J Gen Med. 2024;17:5417–22.
4. Lillicrap TP, Santoro A, Marris L, Akerman CJ, Hinton G. Backpropagation and the brain. Nat Rev Neurosci. 2020;21(6):335–46.
5. González P, Castaño A, Chawla NV, Coz JJD. A review on quantification learning. ACM Comput Surv. 2017;50(5):Article 74.
6. Hartrick CT, Kovan JP, Shapiro S. The numeric rating scale for clinical pain measurement: a ratio measure? Pain Pract. 2003;3(4):310–6.
7. Williamson A, Hoggart B. Pain: a review of three commonly used pain rating scales. J Clin Nurs. 2005;14(7):798–804.
8. Santos CFGD, Papa JP. Avoiding overfitting: a survey on regularization methods for convolutional neural networks. ACM Comput Surv. 2022;54(10s):Article 213.
9. Liu Y, Primiero CA, Kulkarni V, Soyer HP, Betz-Stablein B. Artificial intelligence for the classification of pigmented skin lesions in populations with skin of color: a systematic review. Dermatology. 2023;239(4):499–513.
10. Ganaie MA, Hu M, Malik AK, Tanveer M, Suganthan PN. Ensemble deep learning: a review. Eng Appl Artif Intell. 2022;115:105151.
11. Radcliffe K, Lyson HC, Barr-Walker J, Sarkar U. Collective intelligence in medical decision-making: a systematic scoping review. BMC Med Inform Decis Mak. 2019;19(1):158.
12. Blanchard MD, Herzog SM, Kämmer JE, Zöller N, Kostopoulou O, Kurvers RHJM. Collective intelligence increases diagnostic accuracy in a general practice setting. Med Decis Mak. 2024;44(4):451–62.
13. Barnett ML, Boddupalli D, Nundy S, Bates DW. Comparative accuracy of diagnosis by collective intelligence of multiple physicians vs individual physicians. JAMA Netw Open. 2019;2(3):e190096–e.
14. Specchia ML, Frisicale EM, Carini E, Di Pilla A, Cappa D, Barbara A, et al. The impact of tumor board on cancer care: evidence from an umbrella review. BMC Health Serv Res. 2020;20(1):73.
15. O'Leary KJ, Wayne DB, Haviley C, Slade ME, Lee J, Williams MV. Improving teamwork: impact of structured interdisciplinary rounds on a medical teaching unit. J Gen Intern Med. 2010;25(8):826–32.
16. Agarwal N, Sondhi A, Chopra K, Singh G. Transfer learning: survey and classification. In: Smart Innovations in Communication and Computational Sciences: Proceedings of ICSICCS 2020; 2021. p. 145–55.
17. Yosinski J, Clune J, Bengio Y, Lipson H. How transferable are features in deep neural networks? Adv Neural Inf Process Syst. 2014;27
18. Deng C, Ji X, Rainey C, Zhang J, Lu W. Integrating machine learning with human knowledge. iScience. 2020;23(11):101656.
19. Tsiknakis N, Theodoropoulos D, Manikis G, Ktistakis E, Boutsora O, Berto A, et al. Deep learning for diabetic retinopathy detection and classification based on fundus images: a review. Comput Biol Med. 2021;135:104599.
20. Gutierrez AN, Halvorsen PH, Rong Y. MBA degree is needed for leadership roles in medical physics profession. J Appl Clin Med Phys. 2017;18(6):6–9.
21. Ackerly DC, Sangvai DG, Udayakumar K, Shah BR, Kalman NS, Cho AH, et al. Training the next generation of physician–executives: an innovative residency pathway in management and leadership. Acad Med. 2011;86(5):575–9.
22. Wu J, Gu N. New orientation of Interdisciplinarity in medicine: engineering medicine. Engineering. 2024;45:252–61.
23. Baturalp TB, Bozkurt S, Baldock C. The future of biomedical engineering education is transdisciplinary. Phys Eng Sci Med. 2024;47:779–82.

24. Weerarathna IN, Kumar P, Luharia A, Mishra G. Engineering with biomedical sciences changing the horizon of healthcare-a review. Bioengineered. 2024;15(1):2401269.
25. Poskett J. Horizons: a global history of science. London, UK: Penguin UK; 2022.
26. Sendi P, Gafni A, Birch S. Ethical economics and cost–effectiveness analysis: is it ethical to ignore opportunity costs? Expert Rev Pharmacoecon Outcomes Res. 2005;5(6):661–5.
27. Perkmann M, Tartari V, McKelvey M, Autio E, Broström A, D'Este P, et al. Academic engagement and commercialisation: a review of the literature on university–industry relations. Res Policy. 2013;42(2):423–42.
28. Suzuki K. Overview of deep learning in medical imaging. Radiol Phys Technol. 2017;10(3):257–73.
29. Mouton CP, Bazaldua OV, Pierce B, Espino DV. Common infections in older adults. Am Fam Physician. 2001;63(2):257–68.
30. Malone ML, Gennis V, Goodwin JS. Characteristics of diabetic ketoacidosis in older versus younger adults. J Am Geriatr Soc. 1992;40(11):1100–4.
31. Ramanujam VS, Anderson KE. Porphyria diagnostics-part 1: a brief overview of the Porphyrias. Curr Protoc Hum Genet. 2015;86:17.20.1–6.
32. Thomson H, Francis DM. Abdominal-wall tenderness: a useful sign in the acute abdomen. Lancet. 1977;2(8047):1053–4.
33. Li H, Klabjan D. Reverse Prompt Engineering arXiv preprint arXiv:241106729. 2024.
34. Mamede S, Schmidt HG. Reflection in medical diagnosis: a literature review. Health Professions Education. 2017;3(1):15–25.
35. Sandars J. The use of reflection in medical education: AMEE guide no. 44. Med Teach. 2009;31(8):685–95.
36. Mann K, Gordon J, MacLeod A. Reflection and reflective practice in health professions education: a systematic review. Adv Health Sci Educ. 2009;14(4):595–621.

Understanding Core AI Concepts

8

Abstract

Artificial intelligence has revolutionized the field of medical diagnostics, offering tools and techniques that enhance accuracy, efficiency, and patient care. This chapter provides an understanding of the core artificial intelligence concepts, including human intelligence versus artificial intelligence, machine learning, deep learning, artificial neural networks, convolutional neural networks, large language models, and natural language processing. These technologies form the backbone of modern artificial intelligence applications in health care.

Keywords

Human intelligence · Machine learning · Neural networks · Convolutional neural networks · Recurrent neural networks · Large language models · Natural language processing · Prompt engineering

8.1 Human Intelligence Versus Artificial Intelligence

Human intelligence refers to the cognitive capabilities of humans, encompassing reasoning, problem-solving, learning, memory, and emotional understanding. These capabilities allow us to perform complex tasks, adapt to changing environments, and make decisions informed by intuition and ethical considerations.

On the other hand, artificial intelligence refers to the development of computational systems that attempt to emulate certain aspects of human cognition [1]. These systems leverage algorithms, data structures, and machine learning models to process information, recognize patterns, and solve problems. For example, large language models can generate human-like language based on probabilistic regularities and distributional relationships in vast datasets [2]. However, unlike humans, these models do not draw on lived experience, contextual awareness, or intrinsic understanding. Their outputs are shaped by likelihood estimations across patterns in data,

T. Hirosawa, *Artificial Intelligence in Medical Diagnostics*,
https://doi.org/10.1007/978-981-95-4338-0_8

rather than by an integrated cognitive framework or intentional meaning-making. While artificial intelligence can mimic specific cognitive tasks with high accuracy and efficiency, it fundamentally differs from human intelligence in its origins, architecture, cognitive mechanisms, and range of application.

8.1.1 Origins and Structural Differences

Human intelligence is biological, developed over millions of years for evolution. It reflects adaptability, emotional comprehension, and social cooperation. In contrast, artificial intelligence is an engineered system, built using silicon-based hardware and programming languages. Structurally, the human brain is an intricate network of carbon-based neurons capable of parallel processing, allowing for flexible, abstract thinking and emotional awareness. Conversely, artificial intelligence systems rely on digital processors and artificial neural networks that follow defined algorithms or learn from large datasets.

8.1.2 Cognitive Process and Reasoning

The thinking processes inherent to human intelligence involve abstract reasoning, emotional intuition, creativity, and the capacity to understand ethical dilemmas through subjective experience. These capabilities empower humans to navigate ambiguous or complex situations effectively. Artificial intelligence systems, however, operate on algorithmically driven logic, pattern recognition, and statistical inference, limiting their ability to understand contexts beyond their training datasets or to intuitively grasp nuances without explicit programming.

8.1.3 Adaptability, Cultural Learning, and Contextual Understanding

Human intelligence exhibits superior adaptability by applying creativity, emotional thought, and ethical reasoning to complex scenarios. Artificial intelligence, while efficient in data-driven tasks, operates within fixed parameters by the constraints of its programming and training data. Furthermore, human intelligence benefits from cultural transmission and experiential learning across generations. This allows for nuanced understanding of social norms, ethics, and collective knowledge. Artificial intelligence systems, though capable of processing large datasets rapidly, lack the lived experience and social learning mechanisms that provide humans with cultural depth and moral perspective.

These differences highlight the collaborative potential of human and artificial intelligence in medical diagnostics, where artificial intelligence systems augment human expertise rather than replace it [3]. Because of these fundamental differences, some writers have referred to "AI" as "Alien Intelligence," highlighting its potentially unfamiliar and divergent nature from human cognition [4, 5].

8.1.4 Implications for Medical Diagnostics

Given these differences, artificial intelligence should be viewed as augmenting rather than replacing human intelligence in medical diagnostics. Artificial intelligence excels at analyzing complex datasets, identifying patterns, and supporting clinical decisions with speed and precision. However, health-care professionals contribute indispensable qualities: empathy, ethical judgment, and contextual insight. The most effective diagnostic systems combine the analytical strengths of artificial intelligence with the humane expertise of health-care professionals.

The concept of "hybrid intelligence," explored further in Chap. 15, emphasizes the synergy between human and artificial cognition. Such collaboration holds the potential to enhance diagnostic accuracy, efficiency, and patient care outcomes. The key differences between human and artificial intelligence are summarized in Table 8.1.

Table. 8.1 Key differences between human and artificial intelligence

Feature	Artificial intelligence	Human intelligence
Origin	Human design	Biological evolution
Time span	Decades for development	Millions of years for evolution
Basis	Processing units, algorithms, data	Carbon-based, organic brain
Consciousness	Lacks consciousness and subjective experience	Possesses consciousness and subjective experience
Thinking style	Pattern recognition, statistical analysis, logical reasoning	Intuitive, conceptual, emotional, common sense reasoning
Learning	Specialized, data-driven learning	Generalpurpose, experiential learning
Embodiment	Disembodied; interaction mainly via robotics	Embodied; shaped by physical interaction
Biases	Biases from training data and algorithms	Cognitive biases
Decision-making	Programmed logic and optimization; can be transparent or a "black box"	Influenced by intuition and emotions; can be transparent or opaque
Goals	Programmed objectives; potential for emergent goals	Driven by biological needs, social factors, and personal desires
Evolution	Rapid, iterative development and self-improvement	Slow, generational biological changes
Creativity	Domain-specific outputs derived from data patterns	Novel ideas and concepts across diverse domains
Limitations	Superior processing speed, storage, and endurance; lacks fatigue	Limited processing speed and memory; subject to fatigue and physical limits
Understanding of the world	Limited common-sense reasoning and contextual understanding	Holistic understanding; cause-and-effect reasoning from experience
Values and ethics	Requires explicit programming; risk of bias if poorly designed	Innate moral and ethical frameworks influenced by culture and society

Recognizing and respecting the fundamental differences between human and artificial intelligence is crucial. Thoughtful integration, guided by ethical design and sustained human oversight, is essential to harness the full potential of artificial intelligence in medical diagnostics while preserving the human-centered values at the core of health care.

8.2 Machine Learning

While the broad field of artificial intelligence, machine learning represents a subset of techniques that enables systems to learn from data without being explicitly programmed. Deep learning is, in turn, a specialized and powerful type of machine learning that uses complex neural networks to mimic human decision-making processes. In essence, machine learning focuses on algorithms that learn from data, whereas deep learning uses complex neural networks to mimic human decision-making processes. In medical diagnostics, machine learning algorithms analyze vast datasets, identify patterns, and make predictions to support health-care professionals in decision-making. Deep learning, through its neural network structures, excels at tasks like medical image analysis and natural language understanding, often enhancing the performance of traditional machine learning techniques. The primary goal of these artificial intelligence-driven approaches in medical diagnostics is to improve diagnostic accuracy, reduce human error, and optimize treatment planning. Machine learning techniques in medical diagnostics include supervised learning, which uses labeled data to train models for predictions such as disease detection. Unsupervised learning identifies hidden patterns in unlabeled data, for example, clustering patients with similar symptoms, while reinforcement learning focuses on decision-making in dynamic environments, such as robotic surgeries or personalized treatment plans [6].

8.2.1 Common Machine Learning Methods

Machine learning encompasses a variety of methods, each with its unique applications and strengths [7]. Some widely used methods include the following:

- K-Means Clustering: This is an unsupervised learning algorithm used for grouping data into clusters based on their similarities. In medical diagnostics, it can help identify patterns in patient data, such as grouping individuals with similar symptoms or risk factors, as shown in Fig. 8.1.
- Logistic Regression: A supervised learning algorithm used for binary classification tasks. It is commonly applied in predicting the likelihood of a patient having a specific condition based on diagnostic metrics.
- Linear Regression: This method predicts continuous outcomes, such as estimating a patient's blood pressure based on various health parameters [8], as shown in Fig. 8.2.

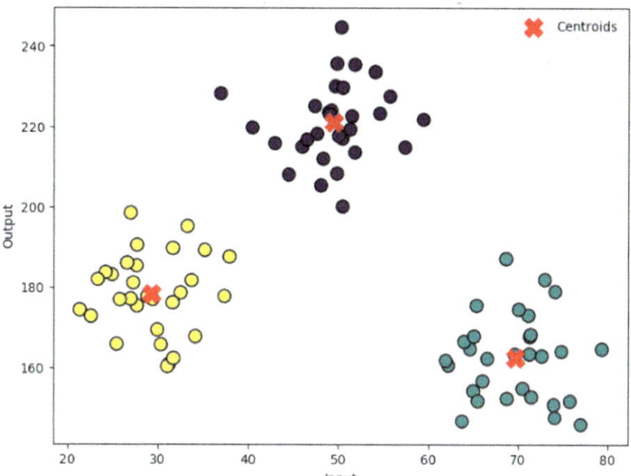

Fig. 8.1 Example for K-means clustering

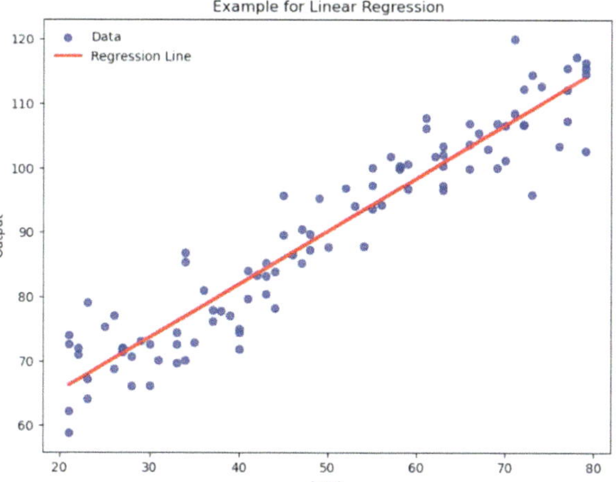

Fig. 8.2 Example for linear regression model

- Decision Trees: These are simple yet powerful tools for classification and regression tasks [9]. In health care, decision trees can help map out diagnostic pathways and treatment recommendations [10].
- Random Forests: An ensemble learning method that builds multiple decision trees and combines their outputs for improved accuracy. By averaging the predictions of many trees, this method reduces the risk of overfitting and often achieves better generalization than a single tree. It is particularly useful for handling complex datasets in medical diagnostics, such as predicting disease outcomes from diverse health variables.

These methods provide a foundational toolkit for building artificial intelligence systems in health care, enabling robust and efficient analysis of medical data.

8.2.2 Artificial Neural Networks

Artificial neural networks are at the core of machine learning techniques used in medical diagnostics. Inspired by the structure and functioning of the human brain, they consist of layers of interconnected nodes, often called artificial neurons, that are inspired by the structure and functioning of the human brain. These neural networks are capable of learning complex relationships in data by adjusting the weights through training processes. Artificial neural networks are widely applied in medical diagnostics for tasks such as disease classification, where they classify diseases based on medical imaging data like X-rays, computed tomography scans, or magnetic resonance imaging [11]. They are also used for patient risk prediction, analyzing patient history and health parameters to predict the likelihood of disease progression, and for signal analysis, particularly in interpreting electrocardiography and electroencephalogram data to detect abnormalities [12, 13]. For example, an artificial neural network trained on magnetic resonance imaging brain images can successfully differentiate between tumors and normal tissues, aiding in early detection of cancer [14]. The representative subtype of artificial neural networks, such as conventional neural networks and recurrent neural networks, are introduced in the following Sects. 8.2.3 and 8.2.4.

8.2.3 Convolutional Neural Networks

Convolutional neural networks are specialized artificial neural networks designed for processing data with a grid-like method, such as images. Convolutional neural networks excel at feature extraction and pattern recognition, making them indispensable in medical imaging analysis. The key components of convolutional neural networks include convolutional layers, which extract spatial features from input images using filters; pooling layers, which reduce the dimensionality of features while retaining essential information; and fully connected layers, which combine the extracted features for final classification or prediction [15]. Convolutional neural networks are widely used in medical diagnostics for tasks such as image recognition to detect fractures, tumors, or lesions from X-rays and magnetic resonance imaging, retinal disease detection to identify diabetic retinopathy from fundus images, and cancer detection for automating the early detection of breast cancer from mammograms [16, 17]. For instance, a convolutional neural network-based model trained on chest X-ray datasets can accurately detect pneumonia with performance metrics surpassing those of human radiologists [18].

8.2.4 Recurrent Neural Networks

Recurrent neural networks are another important class of artificial neural networks designed for processing sequential data, making them particularly effective for analyzing time-dependent information. While convolutional neural networks excel at spatial feature extraction in images, recurrent neural networks are designed to handle temporal relationships in data, such as signals or text sequences. Recurrent neural networks are equipped with a feedback loop that allows information to persist across time steps, which enables them to model dependencies between previous and current inputs [19].

In medical diagnostics, recurrent neural networks play a significant role in applications where time series data or sequential inputs are analyzed. For example, recurrent neural networks are used to process electrocardiogram and electroencephalogram signals to detect abnormalities, predict disease progression, and monitor patient health over time [12, 13]. They are also applied in medical text analysis to understand sequential information in clinical notes, such as identifying the chronology of treatments or patient histories [20]. Although recurrent neural networks have certain limitations, such as difficulty handling long-term dependencies, these have been addressed by more advanced variants like long short-term memory networks and gated recurrent units, which enhance their ability to retain information over extended sequences.

Together, convolutional neural networks and recurrent neural networks form complementary tools in medical diagnostics, with convolutional neural networks focusing on spatial data and recurrent neural networks excelling at temporal or sequential data. This combined capability is critical in building robust artificial intelligence systems that can analyze both static images and dynamic information effectively.

8.3 Large Language Models

Large language models are advanced artificial intelligence systems trained on massive text datasets to process, generate, and analyze human language. These models are crucial in processing unstructured clinical data, such as physician notes, research publications, and electronic health records. Large language models leverage billions of parameters and are built on architectures like transformers, which capture contextual relationships within textual information. In medical diagnostics, they have the potential to enhance documentation, extract insights, and improve clinical decision support [21].

8.3.1 Natural Language Processing

Natural language processing is a branch of artificial intelligence that focuses on the interaction between computers and human language. Natural language processing provides the foundational techniques that enable large language models to process text data effectively. While natural language processing focuses on specific tasks such as text analysis, speech recognition, and language generation, large language models represent an advanced implementation of natural language processing, leveraging massive datasets and architectures like transformers to achieve state-of-the-art performance [22].

Transformers are artificial neural network architectures designed to handle sequential data efficiently by using self-attention mechanisms to understand contextual relationships within text [23]. This allows transformers to process long and complex medical documents with remarkable accuracy and speed, making them highly valuable for users, including health-care professionals [24]. In the medical field, natural language processing techniques facilitate processes such as clinical text summarization, where lengthy electronic health records are condensed to present key findings to health-care professionals; medical coding automation, which translates clinical narratives into standardized codes for billing and insurance purposes; and information extraction, which identifies symptoms, diseases, and treatments from physician notes. For example, natural language processing models can analyze unstructured clinical notes to identify mentions of symptoms, drug prescriptions, and potential adverse events, ultimately improving patient safety [22].

8.3.2 Tokenization

The term "token" carries historical connotations, having previously referred to traditional forms of currency predating modern paper and coin systems [25]. In the context of natural language processing, it has acquired a distinct meaning. Tokenization is a fundamental step in natural language processing where textual data is broken down into smaller units, called tokens [26]. These tokens serve as the building blocks on which large language models operate, enabling them to effectively process and to generate text outputs. Critically, the number of tokens processed both as input and generated as output directly impacts computational resources and, consequently, the cost associated with using large language models. Users often face constraints in the form of maximum token limits or pay-per-token pricing models.

Tokenization can be performed at various levels. Word-level tokenization splits text into words; subword tokenization breaks words into meaningful subcomponents, such as breaking the word "diagnostic" into "diagnos" and "tic"; and character-level tokenization splits text into individual characters. For example, the input text "AI improves medical diagnostics" can be tokenized at the word level into ["AI," "improves," "medical," "diagnostics," "."] or at the subword level into ["AI," "improve," "s," "medical," "diagnostic," "s"]. In medical diagnostics, tokenization enables large language models to process clinical texts efficiently, ensuring accurate representation and analysis of data [27].

8.3.3 Vectorization

These tokens are transformed into numerical representations that can be understood by machine learning models. This step is essential for bridging the gap between human-readable text and mathematical operations used by artificial intelligence systems [20]. In medical diagnostics, tokenization and vectorization enable large language models to process clinical texts efficiently, ensuring accurate representation and analysis of data [28].

8.3.4 Prompt

A new concept closely tied to natural language processing and large language models is the use of "prompts." Prompts are system instructions or queries that guide artificial intelligence models like large language models to generate specific and relevant outputs. Unlike system instructions, often referred to as a system prompt, which dictate overarching operational rules for an artificial intelligence, prompts serve as contextual inputs that elicit responses tailored to specific tasks or questions.

Prompt engineering is a critical aspect of utilizing artificial intelligence effectively, particularly in domains like medical diagnostics. This practice involves carefully designing and optimizing prompts to elicit highly relevant and accurate outputs from artificial intelligence systems such as large language models [29]. Reversed prompt engineering, which involves analyzing artificial intelligence outputs to infer the original prompts, is discussed in Sect. 7.10. This method provides complementary insights into prompt behavior and model interaction. For instance, a study reported that when large language models were tested against medical benchmarks using various prompts, including "think step by step," a 1–2% improvement in performance was observed [30]. By leveraging prompt engineering, future health-care professionals can fine-tune artificial intelligence behavior to meet specific diagnostic needs, such as summarizing patient records or generating insights from complex research data.

8.3.5 Adjustable Parameters

Prompt engineering involves designing and optimizing prompts by adjusting several parameters to elicit highly relevant and accurate outputs [31]. These adjustable parameters include temperature, which controls the randomness or creativity of the model's output. Temperature controls the randomness of the output, where higher values (0.7–1.0) increase diversity, while lower values (0.0–0.3) produce focused, deterministic results.

Top P, also referred to as nucleus sampling, limits the range of word choices by selecting the smallest set of words whose cumulative probability exceeds a specified threshold, for instance, 0.9. This parameter is often used in conjunction with temperature to balance creativity and coherence effectively. For example, a higher Top *P* value allows for a broader range of word selection, whereas a lower value ensures focused and relevant outputs.

Max token length defines the maximum number of tokens in the generated response, helping tailor outputs to specific tasks such as concise summaries or detailed explanations. Additionally, safety settings ensure outputs align with ethical and domain-specific requirements, critical for sensitive fields like medical diagnostics. By effectively tuning these parameters, health-care professionals can optimize artificial intelligence systems for precise, context-aware, and reliable outputs tailored to their diagnostic needs.

In summary, this chapter outlines the foundational artificial intelligence concepts essential for understanding modern medical diagnostics. It highlights machine learning, artificial neural networks, convolutional neural networks, large language models, and natural language processing, emphasizing their practical applications and transformative impact on health care. As artificial intelligence continues to evolve, its role in medical diagnostics will only become more significant, offering improved outcomes for both patients and health-care professionals.

References

1. Spector JM, Ma S. Inquiry and critical thinking skills for the next generation: from artificial intelligence back to human intelligence. Smart Learn Environ. 2019;6(1):1–11.
2. Chang Y, Wang X, Wang J, Wu Y, Yang L, Zhu K, et al. A survey on evaluation of large language models. ACM Trans Intell Syst Technol. 2024;15(3):1–45.
3. Karches KE. Against the iDoctor: why artificial intelligence should not replace physician judgment. Theor Med Bioeth. 2018;39(2):91–110.
4. Harari YN. Nexus: a brief history of information networks from the stone age to AI. Random House; 2024.
5. Martin J. Alien intelligence. J Bus Strategy. 2001;22(2):18–23.
6. Delipetrev B, Tsinaraki, C. and Kostic, U. Historical evolution of artificial intelligence. Luxembourg: Publications Office of the European Union; 2020.
7. Lilly CM, Soni AV, Dunlap D, Hafer N, Picard MA, Buchholz B, et al. Advancing point-of-care testing by application of machine learning techniques and artificial intelligence. Chest. 2025;167(1):152–9.
8. Skrepnek GH. Regression methods in the empiric analysis of health care data. J Manag Care Pharm. 2005;11(3):240–51.
9. Kingsford C, Salzberg SL. What are decision trees? Nat Biotechnol. 2008;26(9):1011–3.
10. Podgorelec V, Kokol P, Stiglic B, Rozman I. Decision trees: an overview and their use in medicine. J Med Syst. 2002;26:445–63.
11. Anwar SM, Majid M, Qayyum A, Awais M, Alnowami M, Khan MK. Medical image analysis using convolutional neural networks: a review. J Med Syst. 2018;42(11):226.
12. Moreno-Sánchez PA, García-Isla G, Corino VDA, Vehkaoja A, Brukamp K, van Gils M, et al. ECG-based data-driven solutions for diagnosis and prognosis of cardiovascular diseases: a systematic review. Comput Biol Med. 2024;172:108235.
13. Amer NS, Belhaouari SB. EEG signal processing for medical diagnosis, healthcare, and monitoring: a comprehensive review. IEEE Access. 2023;11:143116–42.
14. Solanki S, Singh UP, Chouhan SS, Jain S. Brain tumor detection and classification using intelligence techniques: an overview. IEEE Access. 2023;11:12870–86.
15. Li Z, Liu F, Yang W, Peng S, Zhou J. A survey of convolutional neural networks: analysis, applications, and prospects. IEEE Trans Neural Networks Learn Syst. 2021;33(12):6999–7019.
16. Tsiknakis N, Theodoropoulos D, Manikis G, Ktistakis E, Boutsora O, Berto A, et al. Deep learning for diabetic retinopathy detection and classification based on fundus images: a review. Comput Biol Med. 2021;135:104599.
17. Jairam MP, Ha R. A review of artificial intelligence in mammography. Clin Imaging. 2022;88:36–44.
18. Wassan S, Dongyan H, Suhail B, Jhanjhi NZ, Xiao G, Ahmed S, et al. Deep convolutional neural network and IoT technology for healthcare. Digit Health. 2024;10:20552076231220123.

19. Yu Y, Si X, Hu C, Zhang J. A review of recurrent neural networks: LSTM cells and network architectures. Neural Comput. 2019;31(7):1235–70.
20. Percha B. Modern clinical text mining: a guide and review. Annu Rev Biomed Data Sci. 2021;4(1):165–87.
21. Zhao WX, Zhou K, Li J, Tang T, Wang X, Hou Y, et al. A survey of large language models. arXiv preprint arXiv:230318223. 2023.
22. Zhou B, Yang G, Shi Z, Ma S. Natural language processing for smart healthcare. IEEE Rev Biomed Eng. 2022;17:4–18.
23. Vaswani A, Shazeer N, Parmar N, Uszkoreit J, Jones L, Gomez AN, et al. Attention is all you need. Adv Neural Inf Process Syst. 2017;30:5998–6008.
24. Lin T, Wang Y, Liu X, Qiu X. A survey of transformers. AI Open. 2022;3:111–32.
25. Ezzamel M, Hoskin K. Retheorizing accounting, writing and money with evidence from Mesopotamia and ancient Egypt. Crit Perspect Account. 2002;13(3):333–67.
26. Jurafsky D, Martin J. Speech and language processing. 2nd ed. Englewood Cliffs: Prentice-Hall; 2008.
27. Behera SK, Nayak MM. Natural language processing for text and speech processing: a review paper. Int J Adv Res Eng Technol. 2020;11(11):1947–52.
28. Kalyan KS, Sangeetha S. SECNLP: a survey of embeddings in clinical natural language processing. J Biomed Inform. 2020;101:103323.
29. Zaghir J, Naguib M, Bjelogrlic M, Névéol A, Tannier X, Lovis C. Prompt engineering paradigms for medical applications: scoping review. J Med Internet Res. 2024;26:e60501.
30. Liévin V, Hother CE, Motzfeldt AG, Winther O. Can large language models reason about medical questions? Patterns. 2024;5(3):100943.
31. Choi J, Lee B. Accelerating materials language processing with large language models. Commun Mater. 2024;5(1):13.

Case Studies in AI-Enhanced Diagnostics

9

Abstract

This chapter provides insights into the application of artificial intelligence in diagnostic processes through various case studies. The chapter first explores the integration of artificial intelligence into diagnostic methodologies, including its role in differential diagnosis and clinical reasoning. Next, the discussion revisits traditional diagnostic techniques, such as the physical examination and phonocardiogram, and demonstrates how these methods are enhanced with artificial intelligence. The chapter concludes by examining specific medical domains, including general diagnostic performance, emergency department, radiology, pathology, cardiology, neurology, gastroenterology, psychiatry, telemedicine, and dermatology. These case studies demonstrate both the advantages and the limitations of artificial intelligence-based diagnostics.

Keywords

Differential diagnosis · Clinical reasoning · Diagnostic performance · Radiology · Pathology · Cardiology · Neurology · Telemedicine

9.1 Artificial Intelligence-Enhanced Diagnostics

This section explores the role of artificial intelligence in supporting health-care professionals during the process of differential diagnosis.

9.1.1 Artificial Intelligence in Differential Diagnosis

Artificial intelligence systems analyze extensive datasets, including patient histories, physical examination, and investigation results to identify possible conditions and prioritize them based on statistical likelihood. For example, diagnostic CDSSs

T. Hirosawa, *Artificial Intelligence in Medical Diagnostics*,
https://doi.org/10.1007/978-981-95-4338-0_9

like DXplain® and Isabel Pro have been shown to improve the performance of health-care professionals by aiding in the resolution of diagnostic cases [1, 2]. These tools effectively assist health-care professionals in analyzing complex patient data to arrive at more accurate and timely diagnoses.

Especially for generative artificial intelligence systems, neither of these systems was specially trained or reinforced for medical diagnoses, yet they have demonstrated surprising potential in analyzing medical scenarios. For example, ChatGPT-4, developed by OpenAI, demonstrated comparable performance with Isabel Pro in difficult diagnostic case series [3]. ChatGPT-3.5 and ChatGPT-4's performance in generating differential diagnoses is comparable to that of medical experts retrospectively assessing the same cases in emergency departments [4]. Several research studies have demonstrated that generative artificial intelligence systems show promise in diagnostic performance for diagnostically challenging case series. While ChatGPT-3.5 is no longer in service, it showed better diagnostic performance for mock cases based on common chief concerns [5]. For the case report series, ChatGPT-4 has demonstrated superior diagnostic performance to ChatGPT-3.5 [6] and to other generative artificial intelligence systems [7]. Another example is Gemini, developed by Google AI, which has surpassed Bard, its previous version [8]. Additionally, LLaMA-3, developed by Meta AI, has shown improvements over LLaMA-2 [9]. Furthermore, these generative artificial intelligence systems improve their diagnostic performance with iterative versions, benefiting from rapid advancements in technology. These studies primarily focused on final diagnoses included in the generated differential diagnosis lists. However, there were discrepancies compared to real-world settings, such as disease prevalence and incomplete clinical information. Therefore, further evaluation is necessary to determine their practical application and reliability in clinical settings.

9.1.2 Artificial Intelligence in Clinical Reasoning

Artificial intelligence contributes to clinical reasoning as a decision-support system for solving complex clinical problems. For example, clinical problem-solving style is a valuable method for health-care professionals to learn and train their clinical reasoning skills. While traditional case reports style often reveals the final diagnosis at the beginning and sometimes focuses on treatment or management, clinical problem-solving style focuses on a single case with a difficult diagnosis. Additionally, clinical information is shown step-by-step according to clinical flow. The final diagnosis is typically not revealed until the definitive investigation is performed, and the discussants share their clinical reasoning at each step [10].

These clinical problem-solving exercises are valuable for comparing and contrasting how health-care professionals and generative artificial intelligence systems approach the diagnostic process [11]. For instance, in a case where a patient presents with multiple symptoms—such as fever, cough, and chest pain—a broad range of possible conditions could be responsible. Some symptoms are respiratory, including community-acquired pneumonia, pulmonary embolism, or viral bronchitis. Others may be cardiac in origin, such as pericarditis. In this context, artificial intelligence systems can assist by analyzing these nonspecific presentations, weighing probabilities, and suggesting the most likely differential diagnoses alongside appropriate next steps, such as ordering imaging or laboratory tests. Artificial intelligence not only highlights potential conditions that health-care professionals might otherwise overlook but also reinforces structured, evidence-based reasoning.

This integration of artificial intelligence into clinical reasoning supports health-care professionals by clarifying diagnostic uncertainty, prioritizing investigations, and providing a transparent rationale for decision-making. Ultimately, it fosters more accurate clinical judgments and improves patient outcomes.

9.2 Revisiting Traditional Diagnostic Techniques with Artificial Intelligence

Traditional diagnostic approaches, including history taking, physical examination, and phonocardiogram, were rapidly becoming a lost art due to advancements in medical technologies [12, 13]. This is partly due to investigation-centered clinical practice in current medicine, often conducted without enough history taking and physical examination before performing diagnostic tests [14]. It is further compounded by gaps in medical education, as medical teachers may not adequately train learners in the bedside art of clinical diagnosis [15]. However, a revisitation of these methods has occurred with the emergence of artificial intelligence, as summarized in Table 9.1. The histories of these traditional diagnostic approaches are detailed in Chap. 2.

9.2.1 Revisiting History Taking

History taking has become a lost art due to the shift toward advanced clinical practice [14, 16]. Recent advancements in artificial intelligence are revitalizing history-taking skills by introducing virtual patients powered by large language models.

Table 9.1 Revisiting traditional diagnostic techniques with artificial intelligence (AI)

Technique	Limitation before AI	Resolution through AI
History taking	Often neglected due to focus on investigation-centered clinical practice	AI powered virtual patients that simulate clinical scenarios for practicing communication and reasoning skills
Physical examination	Decline in cardiac auscultation skills due to reliance on advanced imaging techniques	AI-integrated digital stethoscopes analyze body sounds to detect abnormalities, such as aortic stenosis, with high accuracy
Phonocardiogram	Rarely used due to the rise of ultrasound and difficulty in detecting subtle cardiac sounds like S3	AI-enhanced phonocardiograms visualize S3 and other sounds, improving detection of heart failure and valvular abnormalities

These virtual patients simulate clinical scenarios, allowing learners to practice communication and clinical reasoning in a realistic, interactive chatbot interface [17]. The virtual patient scripts cover common presentations, such as chest pain and short of breath. Learners engage with these virtual patients, receiving actionable artificial intelligence-powered feedback on their questioning techniques. This includes identifying well-covered areas and highlighting gaps. Over 45,000 consultations have demonstrated the potential of this approach to enhance skills independently and repeatedly, particularly for complex scenarios like sexual history taking. While challenges such as occasional "hallucinations" and off-topic responses exist, large language models technology offers a scalable, accessible way to supplement traditional clinical training where patient contact is limited [18]. There is potential for these artificial intelligence technologies to enhance history-taking skills of health-care professionals. Training and education for artificial intelligence in health care is discussed in Chap. 14.

9.2.2 Revisiting Physical Examination

Cardiac auscultation, long considered the centerpiece of the physical examination, is rapidly becoming a lost art. The decline of cardiac auscultation has resulted from the widespread availability of advanced imaging techniques, such as echocardiography [13]. However, artificial intelligence has redefined the traditional physical examination by integrating advanced tools such as digital stethoscopes [19, 20]. These devices record and visualize internal body sounds, including cardiac sounds, and analyze them using machine learning algorithms to detect abnormalities. For example, an electronic stethoscope utilizes artificial intelligence for diagnosing conditions like aortic valve stenosis. In the study, this tool achieved 86% sensitivity and 100% specificity for moderate to severe aortic stenosis when tested on derivation groups, and similar performance was observed in validation groups [21]. This artificial intelligence-enhanced auscultation tool exemplifies how technology can transform traditional diagnostic methods, ensuring greater precision and early detection of valvular heart diseases.

9.2.3 Revisiting Phonocardiogram

The third heart sound (S3) is particularly important for detecting clinically significant cardiac sounds [22]. The specificity of S3 is notably high for detecting heart failure in patients presenting with dyspnea, making its identification critical for timely intervention [23]. The phonocardiogram can visualize cardiac sounds, including S3, providing clearer diagnostic insights and enabling health-care professionals to identify early signs of heart failure or other cardiac abnormalities more effectively [24, 25], shown in Fig. 9.1. Though the phonocardiogram had almost been lost due to the development of ultrasound technology, it is being revitalized by the recent technology advancements, including telemedicine, digital stethoscope,

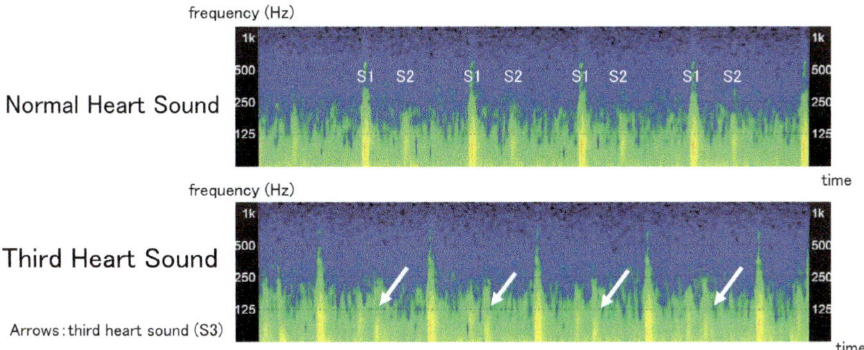

Fig. 9.1 Image of phonocardiogram to visualize the third heart sound (S3)

and artificial intelligence [26, 27]. Machine learning algorithms analyze cardiopulmonary sound recordings for classification. For example, our pilot study developed a machine learning-based system using cardiopulmonary sound files preprocessed through neural network layers. When tested with junior residents, the intervention group adding the machine learning system with remote auscultation demonstrated significantly higher accuracy in identifying normal or abnormal sounds compared to remote auscultation methods (95% vs. 89%, P = 0.003). Though the diagnostic performance for S3 increased by 20%, this improvement was statistically insignificant. This study highlights how machine learning systems enhance early-career healthcare professionals' diagnostic skills, improving accuracy in cardiopulmonary auscultation and supporting accurate screening [28].

9.3 Specific Domains

This section provides domain-specific diagnostic performance by artificial intelligence. The diagnostic performance depends on the dataset, artificial intelligence algorithms, and the evaluation methods.

9.3.1 General Diagnostic Performance

For general diagnostic performance, studies have shown that Isabel Pro produced 175 correct diagnoses (87%) and ChatGPT-4 achieved 165 correct diagnoses (82%) out of 201 difficult complex cases, highlighting the strong potential of artificial intelligence systems in handling challenging diagnostic scenarios [3]. Another study involving 392 case report series revealed that the inclusion rates of the final diagnosis within the top 10 differential diagnosis lists were 87% for ChatGPT-4, 69% for Gemini, and 55% for LLaMA2 chatbot. Furthermore, the top diagnoses matched the final diagnoses in 55% for ChatGPT-4, 31% for Gemini, and 23% for LLaMA2 chatbot, demonstrating ChatGPT-4's higher diagnostic accuracy compared to the others [7]. It is important to note that Isabel Pro has been developed as a diagnostic clinical decision support system, whereas generative AI models such as ChatGPT, Gemini, and LLaMA are not trained or specified for clinical use [29]. Therefore, these findings should be interpreted cautiously as research outcomes rather than clinical recommendations.

9.3.2 Emergency Department

In a retrospective study conducted within an emergency department setting, ChatGPT-4 and ChatGPT-3.5 were evaluated on their ability to generate the top five differential diagnoses both before and after additional investigation. The evaluation was based on 30 anonymized medical charts from the emergency department, focusing solely on text data such as medical history and physical examination findings. Physicians served as the comparison group. Before the inclusion of laboratory investigations, ChatGPT-4 correctly included the definitive diagnosis in the top five differentials in 87% of cases, ChatGPT-3.5 achieved 77%, and physicians reached 83%. After reviewing laboratory results, ChatGPT-4 maintained its 87% accuracy, ChatGPT-3.5 improved significantly to 97%, and physicians achieved an accuracy of 87% [4]. The study's findings highlighted the potential of generative artificial intelligence models, specifically ChatGPT-3.5 and ChatGPT-4, to perform at a level comparable to trained health-care professionals in the task of generating differential diagnoses. Importantly, it should be noted that ChatGPT-3.5 has since been terminated from service, further emphasizing the transient nature of such AI tools. Despite the promising results, these outcomes are intended solely for research purposes. The use of ChatGPT in clinical decision-making should be approached with caution, as the models lack specialized medical training, contextual awareness, and the necessities of clinical decision-making for patient care. Again, generative artificial intelligence models such as ChatGPT-series are not trained or specified for diagnostic purposes. Therefore, these results should be interpreted cautiously as research purposes rather than real-world medical recommendations.

9.3.3 Radiology

Artificial intelligence has become a cornerstone in radiology by enhancing the analysis of imaging studies such as X-rays, computed tomography scans, and magnetic resonance imaging. In one case, artificial intelligence systems detected pulmonary tuberculosis from X-rays in endemic areas, providing radiologists with accurate and actionable insights [30]. These systems are particularly valuable in addressing the growing shortage of radiologists [31] by improving efficiency and ensuring timely diagnoses. For instance, artificial intelligence systems have demonstrated superior performance in detecting breast cancer in mammograms compared to traditional methods, achieving reduced false positives, improved sensitivity, and nearly a 7% increase in the area under the curve, enabling earlier intervention [32]. Other artificial intelligence systems have shown strong performance in detecting pulmonary tuberculosis in chest X-rays, achieving 97% accuracy, 99% area under the curve, 92% sensitivity, and 98% specificity on multiclass classification datasets [30].

9.3.4 Pathology

In pathology, artificial intelligence aids in the microscopic analysis of tissue samples. By identifying abnormal cellular patterns, such as those seen in malignant tumors, artificial intelligence systems have accelerated the diagnostic process and improved accuracy. For instance, in the milestone CAMELYON16 challenge for whole-slide image classification, the best artificial intelligence algorithm achieved an impressive area under the curve of 99%, significantly outperforming pathologists in a diagnostic simulation [33]. This highlights artificial intelligence's potential to enhance accuracy and efficiency in pathological assessments.

9.3.5 Cardiology

Beyond cardiac auscultation and phonocardiogram, artificial intelligence has revolutionized cardiology by improving the interpretation of diagnostic studies, such as electrocardiograms and echocardiograms. A notable case involves the detection of atrial fibrillation through artificial intelligence analysis of heart rhythm data, leading to timely treatment and reduced risk of complications [34, 35]. Additionally, Eleznik et al. developed a deep learning system based on fully convolutional networks that can automatically and precisely predict the occurrence of heart events by measuring the amount and distribution of coronary calcium. In their study involving 20,084 individuals, the system achieved an impressive intraclass correlation coefficient of 0.99, highlighting its potential for accurate cardiovascular risk assessment [36].

9.3.6 Neurology

In neurology, artificial intelligence systems are instrumental in diagnosing neurodegenerative diseases. For example, early-stage Alzheimer's disease was diagnosed in a patient by analyzing imaging biomarkers and cognitive assessment data using advanced machine learning techniques, facilitating early intervention. Additionally, artificial intelligence and machine learning have shown promise in headache research, with applications in natural language processing for structuring clinical data, classification of headache disorders based on neuroimaging and clinical records, and forecasting headaches using self-reported triggers and wearable sensor data. Artificial intelligence is also being explored for predicting treatment responses and optimizing headache management. A review showed that the most common application of machine learning in headache research is classification of headache disorders, typically based on clinical record or neuroimaging data, with accuracies ranging from around 60% to well over 90% [37]. Despite these promising advancements, challenges such as poor reporting and lack of validation in clinical settings remain.

9.3.7 Gastroenterology

Artificial intelligence has enhanced the diagnosis of gastrointestinal disorders through advanced imaging and data analysis. For instance, capsule endoscopy equipped with artificial intelligence algorithms identified small bowel bleeding sources in a patient, providing a definitive diagnosis and guiding effective treatment. Moreover, a systematic analysis demonstrated that artificial intelligence systems with real-time computer-aided polyp detection achieved a significantly higher adenoma detection rate compared to traditional methods (37% versus 25%; $P < 0.01$), highlighting artificial intelligence's role in supporting gastroenterologists with immediate decision-making during procedures [38].

9.3.8 Psychiatry

Artificial intelligence tools in psychiatry analyze speech and behavioral patterns to detect mental health conditions. In one case, natural language processing algorithms identified depressive symptoms in a patient's speech, enabling earlier therapeutic intervention. For example, studies using electroencephalogram-based deep learning methods have demonstrated the ability to distinguish depressive patients from healthy controls with approximately 99% accuracy [39]. While artificial intelligence in psychiatry shows promise, challenges remain, particularly with cultural and linguistic diversity, which can lead to inconsistent diagnostic outcomes. Addressing these limitations requires more diverse training datasets and collaboration with mental health professionals to refine artificial intelligence tools for psychiatric use [40, 41].

9.3.9 Telemedicine

Artificial intelligence strengthens telemedicine by enabling remote diagnostic capabilities. Four emerging trends in the impact of artificial intelligence for telemedicine are as follows: (1) monitoring of patients, (2) using information technology in health care, (3) use of intelligent assistance and diagnosis, and (4) collaborative information analysis [42]. These trends reflect the broad applicability of artificial intelligence technologies to improve patient care remotely.

A comparative study evaluating eight popular symptom assessment apps and general practitioners using 200 primary care vignettes revealed that while no digital tool outperformed general practitioners, some apps demonstrated promising performance. Specifically, Ada achieved a condition coverage of 99% and top 3 suggestion accuracy of 71%, while safe urgency advice accuracy was comparable to general practitioners at 97% [43]. These results highlight the advancements and iterative improvements of artificial intelligence in telemedicine, particularly in the domain of symptom assessment tools. However, it is essential to emphasize that continuous evaluation and validation are necessary to maintain safety, accuracy, and inclusivity, especially across diverse patient populations.

Several of these artificial intelligence-powered platforms have distinct development backgrounds and technical approaches. Babylon Health, launched in 2013 in the United Kingdom, combines online consultations with artificial intelligence-driven assessments and uses a chatbot for symptom checking. While the specifics of its machine learning architecture remain undisclosed, it is believed to utilize recurrent neural networks and possibly Bayesian networks. Ada Health, initially introduced in New Zealand in 2016, employs an adaptive chatbot that responds dynamically to user input and generates shareable health reports. Buoy Health, developed at Harvard Medical School, is a smart symptom checker that uses natural language processing across tens of thousands of clinical sources. Unlike traditional decision-tree models, Buoy dynamically selects questions to reduce diagnostic uncertainty and reportedly achieves diagnostic accuracy above 90% [44].

Moreover, artificial intelligence applications extend beyond symptom checkers. For instance, in tele-stroke programs, artificial intelligence systems analyze imaging and clinical data to assist neurologists in making prompt treatment decisions for patients experiencing acute strokes [45–48]. Similarly, in tele-intensive care unit platforms, artificial intelligence is utilized to monitor critically ill patients and predict potential complications, allowing for timely interventions and enhancing the quality of care delivered in remote or resource-limited settings [49].

9.3.10 Dermatology

Early detection of skin cancer is crucial to prevent mortality and reduce unnecessary invasive procedures [50]. A systematic review revealed that artificial intelligence-based algorithms achieved more than 80% area under the curve in the detection of melanoma [51]. Another systematic review showed that the average accuracy of artificial intelligence applied to detect non-melanoma skin cancer was 87% [52]. These findings highlight artificial intelligence's potential to enhance dermatological diagnostics, improving early detection and clinical decision-making.

In summary of subsection 9.3, domain-specific diagnostic performances by artificial intelligence are detailed in Table 9.2.

In summary, the chapter concludes by synthesizing the insights from the case studies to provide a comprehensive evaluation of artificial intelligence in diagnostics. The analysis emphasizes the remarkable benefits, such as enhanced accuracy, reduced diagnostic time, and improved accessibility to health-care services. However, it also highlights critical limitations, including data bias, issues of interpretability, and the necessity for health-care professionals' oversight to ensure

Table 9.2 Representative data for domain-specific diagnostic performance by artificial intelligence

Domain	AI	Diagnostic performance	Reference
General diagnostic performance	Isabel Pro, ChatGPT-4, Gemini, LLaMA2	Isabel pro: 87% (175/201 cases), ChatGPT-4: 82% (165/201 cases), ChatGPT-4 top-10 inclusion: 87%, top diagnosis match: 55%, Gemini: 69% (top-10), 31% (top diagnosis), LLaMA2: 55% (top-10), 23% (top diagnosis)	[3, 7]
Emergency department	ChatGPT-4, ChatGPT-3.5	Before labs: ChatGPT-4: 87%, ChatGPT-3.5: 77%, physicians: 83%; after labs: ChatGPT-4: 87%, ChatGPT-3.5: 97%, physicians: 87%	[4]
Radiology	Various AI Systems	Pulmonary tuberculosis detection: 97% accuracy, 99% AUC, 92% sensitivity, 98% specificity; breast cancer detection: Approximately 7% AUC improvement, reduced false positives, improved sensitivity	[30, 32]
Pathology	AI Algorithms	CAMELYON16 challenge: Best AI achieved 99% AUC, outperforming pathologists	[33]
Cardiology	DL Model	Detection of atrial fibrillation from heart rhythm data; DL system predicted heart events by coronary calcium measurement; study on 20,084 individuals achieved intraclass correlation coefficient of 0.99, indicating high accuracy for risk assessment	[36]
Neurology	ML, NLP, AI systems	Early Alzheimer's detection via imaging biomarkers & cognitive data; headache disorder classification accuracy: 60% to 90%	[37]
Gastrointestinal medicine	AI Algorithms	Capsule endoscopy AI: Identified bleeding sources; artificial intelligence-assisted polyp detection improved adenoma detection rate: 37% vs 25% ($P < 0.01$)	[38]
Psychiatry	NLP, EEG-based AI	NLP identified depressive speech patterns; EEG-based depression classification accuracy ~99%; challenges with cultural/linguistic diversity	[39]
Telemedicine	AI Systems	Four trends: Patient monitoring, health information technology, intelligent assistance, collaborative analysis; tele-stroke programs: AI assists in acute stroke decisions; tele-ICU: AI monitors patients, predicts complications; comparative study: Ada app achieved 99% condition coverage, 71% top 3 accuracy, 97% urgency advice accuracy comarable to general practitioners	[43]
Dermatology	AI Algorithms	Melanoma detection: >80% AUC; non-melanoma skin cancer detection: 87% accuracy	[51, 52]

Note: "Top 10 inclusion" indicates the percentage of cases where the correct final diagnosis appeared within the AI's top 10 suggestions. "Top diagnosis match" indicates the percentage of cases where the AI's single top suggestion was the correct final diagnosis

AI artificial intelligence, *AUC* area under the curve, *DL* deep learning, *EEG* electroencephalogram, *ML* machine learning, *NLP* natural language processing, *ICU* intensive care unit

reliability and safety. These reflections set the stage for the next Chap. 10, which explores in greater depth the inherent limitations of artificial intelligence in diagnostics, offering a focused exploration of the challenges and potential pitfalls that warrant further investigation.

References

1. Martinez-Franco AI, Sanchez-Mendiola M, Mazon-Ramirez JJ, Hernandez-Torres I, Rivero-Lopez C, Spicer T, et al. Diagnostic accuracy in family medicine residents using a clinical decision support system (DXplain): a randomized-controlled trial. Diagnosis (Berl). 2018;5(2):71–6.
2. Sibbald M, Monteiro S, Sherbino J, LoGiudice A, Friedman C, Norman G. Should electronic differential diagnosis support be used early or late in the diagnostic process? A multicentre experimental study of Isabel. BMJ Qual Saf. 2022;31(6):426–33.
3. Bridges JM. Computerized diagnostic decision support systems—a comparative performance study of Isabel Pro vs. ChatGPT4. Diagnosis (Berl). 2024;11:250.
4. Berg HT, van Bakel B, van de Wouw L, Jie KE, Schipper A, Jansen H, et al. ChatGPT and generating a differential diagnosis early in an emergency department presentation. Ann Emerg Med. 2024;83(1):83–6.
5. Hirosawa T, Harada Y, Yokose M, Sakamoto T, Kawamura R, Shimizu T. Diagnostic accuracy of differential-diagnosis lists generated by generative Pretrained transformer 3 Chatbot for clinical vignettes with common chief complaints: a pilot study. Int J Environ Res Public Health. 2023;20(4)
6. Han T, Adams LC, Bressem KK, Busch F, Nebelung S, Truhn D. Comparative analysis of multimodal large language model performance on clinical vignette questions. JAMA. 2024;331(15):1320–1.
7. Hirosawa T, Harada Y, Mizuta K, Sakamoto T, Tokumasu K, Shimizu T. Diagnostic performance of generative artificial intelligences for a series of complex case reports. Digit Health. 2024;10:20552076241265215.
8. Hirosawa T, Harada Y, Tokumasu K, Ito T, Suzuki T, Shimizu T. Comparative study to evaluate the accuracy of differential diagnosis lists generated by Gemini advanced, Gemini, and bard for a case report series analysis: cross-sectional study. JMIR Med Inform. 2024;12:e63010.
9. Hirosawa T, Harada Y, Tokumasu K, Shiraishi T, Suzuki T, Shimizu T. Comparative analysis of diagnostic performance: differential diagnosis lists by LLaMA3 versus LLaMA2 for case reports. JMIR Form Res. 2024;8:e64844.
10. Kassirer JR. Clinical problem-solving–a new feature in the Journal. N Engl J Med. 1992;326(1):60–1.
11. Restrepo D, Rodman A, Abdulnour RE. Conversations on reasoning: large language models in diagnosis. J Hosp Med. 2024;19:731.
12. Bank I, Vliegen HW, Bruschke AV. The 200th anniversary of the stethoscope: can this low-tech device survive in the high-tech 21st century? Eur Heart J. 2016;37(47):3536–43.
13. Chizner MA. Cardiac auscultation: rediscovering the lost art. Curr Probl Cardiol. 2008;33(7):326–408.
14. Schechter GP, Blank LL, Godwin HA, LaCombe MA, Novack DH, Rosse WF. Refocusing on history-taking skills during internal medicine training. Am J Med. 1996;101(2):210–6.
15. Kern DC, Parrino TA, Korst DR. The lasting value of clinical skills. JAMA. 1985;254(1):70–6.
16. Summerton N. The medical history as a diagnostic technology. Br J Gen Pract. 2008;58(549):273–6.
17. White CB, Wendling A, Lampotang S, Lizdas D, Cordar A, Lok B. The role for virtual patients in the future of medical education. Acad Med. 2017;92(1):10–9.

18. Potter L, Jefferies C. Enhancing communication and clinical reasoning in medical education: building virtual patients with generative AI. Future Healthcare J. 2024;11:100043.
19. Kim Y, Hyon Y, Lee S, Woo S-D, Ha T, Chung C. The coming era of a new auscultation system for analyzing respiratory sounds. BMC Pulm Med. 2022;22(1):119.
20. Jani V, Danford DA, Thompson WR, Schuster A, Manlhiot C, Kutty S. The discerning ear: cardiac auscultation in the era of artificial intelligence and telemedicine. Eur Heart J Digital Health. 2021;2(3):456–66.
21. Ghanayim T, Lupu L, Naveh S, Bachner-Hinenzon N, Adler D, Adawi S, et al. Artificial intelligence-based stethoscope for the diagnosis of aortic stenosis. Am J Med. 2022;135(9):1124–33.
22. Silverman M. The third heart sound. In: Walker HK, Hall WD, Hurst JW, editors. Clinical methods: the history, physical, and laboratory examinations. 3rd ed. Boston: Butterworths; 1990.
23. Wang CS, FitzGerald JM, Schulzer M, Mak E, Ayas NT. Does this dyspneic patient in the emergency department have congestive heart failure? JAMA. 2005;294(15):1944–56.
24. Leatham A. Auscultation and phonocardiography: a personal view of the past 40 years. Br Heart J. 1987;57(5):397–403.
25. Watsjold B, Ilgen J, Monteiro S, Sibbald M, Goldberger ZD, Thompson WR, et al. Do you hear what you see? Utilizing phonocardiography to enhance proficiency in cardiac auscultation. Perspect Med Educ. 2021;10(3):148–54.
26. Hirosawa T, Ito T, Harada Y, Ikenoya K, Yokose M, Shimizu T. The utility of phonocardiograms in real-time remote cardiac auscultation using an internet-connected electronic stethoscope: open-label randomized controlled pilot trial. Digit Health. 2023;9:20552076231161945.
27. Reyna MA, Kiarashi Y, Elola A, Oliveira J, Renna F, Gu A, et al. Heart murmur detection from phonocardiogram recordings: The George B. Moody PhysioNet Challenge 2022. PLoS Digit Health. 2023;2(9):e0000324.
28. Hirosawa T, Sakamoto T, Harada Y, Tokumasu K, Shimizu T. Clinical decision support system using a machine learning model to assist simultaneous cardiopulmonary auscultation: open-label randomized controlled trial. Digit Health. 2024;10:20552076241233689.
29. Ren LY. Isabel Pro. J Canad Health Libraries Assoc. 2019;40(2):63–9.
30. Acharya V, Dhiman G, Prakasha K, Bahadur P, Choraria A, M S, et al. AI-assisted tuberculosis detection and classification from chest X-rays using a deep learning normalization-free network model. Comput Intell Neurosci. 2022;2022:2399428.
31. Rimmer A. Radiologist shortage leaves patient care at risk, warns royal college. BMJ. 2017;359:j4683.
32. Jairam MP, Ha R. A review of artificial intelligence in mammography. Clin Imaging. 2022;88:36–44.
33. Bejnordi BE, Veta M, Van Diest PJ, Van Ginneken B, Karssemeijer N, Litjens G, et al. Diagnostic assessment of deep learning algorithms for detection of lymph node metastases in women with breast cancer. JAMA. 2017;318(22):2199–210.
34. Watson X, D'Souza J, Cooper D, Markham R. Artificial intelligence in cardiology: fundamentals and applications. Intern Med J. 2022;52(6):912–20.
35. Alharbi Y. Artificial intelligence in cardiology: present state and prospective directions. J Radiat Res Appl Sci. 2024;17(3):101012.
36. Zeleznik R, Foldyna B, Eslami P, Weiss J, Alexander I, Taron J, et al. Deep convolutional neural networks to predict cardiovascular risk from computed tomography. Nat Commun. 2021;12(1):715.
37. Stubberud A, Langseth H, Nachev P, Matharu MS, Tronvik E. Artificial intelligence and headache. Cephalalgia. 2024;44(8):03331024241268290.
38. Hassan C, Spadaccini M, Iannone A, Maselli R, Jovani M, Chandrasekar VT, et al. Performance of artificial intelligence in colonoscopy for adenoma and polyp detection: a systematic review and meta-analysis. Gastrointest Endosc. 2021;93(1):77–85.e6.
39. Saeedi A, Saeedi M, Maghsoudi A, Shalbaf A. Major depressive disorder diagnosis based on effective connectivity in EEG signals: a convolutional neural network and long short-term memory approach. Cogn Neurodyn. 2021;15(2):239–52.

40. Chen ZS, Kulkarni P, Galatzer-Levy IR, Bigio B, Nasca C, Zhang Y. Modern views of machine learning for precision psychiatry. Patterns. 2022;3(11):100602.
41. Ray A, Bhardwaj A, Malik YK, Singh S, Gupta R. Artificial intelligence and psychiatry: an overview. Asian J Psychiatr. 2022;70:103021.
42. Pacis DMM, Subido ED, Bugtai NT, editors. Trends in telemedicine utilizing artificial intelligence. AIP conference proceedings. AIP Publishing; 2018.
43. Gilbert S, Mehl A, Baluch A, Cawley C, Challiner J, Fraser H, et al. How accurate are digital symptom assessment apps for suggesting conditions and urgency advice? A clinical vignettes comparison to GPs. BMJ Open. 2020;10(12):e040269.
44. Ćirković A. Evaluation of four artificial intelligence–assisted self-diagnosis apps on three diagnoses: two-year follow-up study. J Med Internet Res. 2020;22(12):e18097.
45. Wechsler LR, Demaerschalk BM, Schwamm LH, Adeoye OM, Audebert HJ, Fanale CV, et al. Telemedicine quality and outcomes in stroke: a scientific statement for healthcare professionals from the American Heart Association/American Stroke Association. Stroke. 2017;48(1):e3–e25.
46. Lazarus G, Permana AP, Nugroho SW, Audrey J, Wijaya DN, Widyahening IS. Telestroke strategies to enhance acute stroke management in rural settings: a systematic review and meta-analysis. Brain Behav. 2020;10(10):e01787.
47. Ali F, Hamid U, Zaidat O, Bhatti D, Kalia JS. Role of artificial intelligence in TeleStroke: an overview. Front Neurol. 2020;11:559322.
48. Demaerschalk BM, Berg J, Chong BW, Gross H, Nystrom K, Adeoye O, et al. American telemedicine association: Telestroke guidelines. Telemed J E Health. 2017;23(5):376–89.
49. Tang R, Zhang S, Ding C, Zhu M, Gao Y. Artificial intelligence in intensive care medicine: bibliometric analysis. J Med Internet Res. 2022;24(11):e42185.
50. Johansson M, Brodersen J, Jørgensen KJ. Screening for reducing morbidity and mortality in malignant melanoma. Cochrane Database Syst Rev. 2019;6(6):CD012352.
51. Patel RH, Foltz EA, Witkowski A, Ludzik J. Analysis of artificial intelligence-based approaches applied to non-invasive imaging for early detection of melanoma: a systematic review. Cancer. 2023;15(19):4694.
52. Foltz EA, Witkowski A, Becker AL, Latour E, Lim JY, Hamilton A, et al. Artificial intelligence applied to non-invasive imaging modalities in identification of nonmelanoma skin cancer: a systematic review. Cancers (Basel). 2024;16(3):629.

The Limitations of AI in Diagnostics 10

Abstract

This chapter explores the limitations of artificial intelligence in medical diagnostics. It focuses on challenges arising from the dynamic nature of diagnosis, professional adoption, and technological constraints. Diagnosis is a constantly evolving process, which introduces complexities in defining and measuring performance. Additionally, ensuring applicability across diverse populations and adapting to temporal changes in medical knowledge remain persistent issues. By addressing these limitations, all stakeholders can develop strategies to improve the integration and efficacy of artificial intelligence in health care.

Keywords

Diagnostic limitations · Overreliance · Patient-provided information · Black box problem · Biased datasets · Data quality · Data diversity · Generalizability

10.1 Overview of Limitations

Artificial intelligence has revolutionized medical diagnostics by providing levels of accuracy, efficiency, and accessibility previously unimaginable. Nevertheless, significant barriers persist that prevent the full realization of its potential. These barriers are structural, professional, and technical in nature, each presenting unique challenges. This section examines these dimensions to provide a comprehensive understanding of the limitations facing artificial intelligence in diagnostics, as shown in Table 10.1.

T. Hirosawa, *Artificial Intelligence in Medical Diagnostics*,
https://doi.org/10.1007/978-981-95-4338-0_10

Table 10.1 Summary of the limitations of artificial intelligence (AI) in medical diagnostics

Category	Subcategory
Diagnosis-related limitations	Difficulties in defining diagnosis
	Challenges in measuring diagnostic performance
	Individual and population variance
	Dynamic change in diagnosis
User-related limitations	Overreliance on AI outputs
	Inadequate, inaccurate, or incomplete information
	Black box problem
Technical limitations	Challenges in development, including biased datasets, data quality, cost
	Complexity of medical data
	Data protection, privacy, and security
Environmental limitations	Social acceptance, AI maturity, and trust
	Lack of standard international regulations
	Limited infrastructure in low-resource settings
	Cultural and regional adaptability
	Integration with existing workflows
Other limitations	Ethical concerns, including fairness and accountability
	Political and regulatory concerns

10.2 The Limitations Related to Diagnosis

The limitations related to diagnosis highlight challenges in defining, measuring, and generalizing diagnostic performance. Addressing these limitations will not only improve the reliability of artificial intelligence-based diagnostic tools but also ensure their applicability across various populations and evolving medical contexts.

10.2.1 Difficulties in Defining Diagnosis

Diagnosis is a dynamic process that evolves over time, requiring frequent updates and adjustments as additional clinical information becomes available [1]. Iterative processes are essential to refine and redefine diagnostic criteria and approaches, ensuring that they remain relevant and effective in real-world scenarios. However, there is a lack of standardized methods to evaluate clinical decision support systems, including those powered by artificial intelligence [2]. Establishing such standards is critical to ensure their reliability and applicability across diverse medical settings.

10.2.2 Challenges in Measuring Diagnostic Performance

The evaluation of diagnostic performance in medical artificial intelligence systems poses several challenges that heavily depend on specific medical contexts. A fundamental step involves careful selection of cases for evaluation, ensuring these cases reflect the full spectrum of clinical scenarios. Effective case selection requires representation across diverse patient demographics, varying disease severities, and a wide range of clinical complexities. Incorporating cases from various clinical settings, including both rural and urban health-care environments, is essential to validate the robustness and practical applicability of diagnostic systems across diverse contexts.

Moreover, it is crucial to balance the representation of rare and common conditions within datasets to avoid biases that could distort diagnostic accuracy. Reliance on open-source datasets, which may not undergo rigorous validation or standardization, can further complicate this balance. Open-source datasets might not be comprehensive or reflective of actual clinical practice, potentially undermining the validity and generalizability of artificial intelligence systems developed from these resources [3]. With advanced artificial intelligence systems capable of crawling Internet resources, the traceability and accountability of data sources have become more complex.

Equally important is the quality and precision of clinical information used as input data. Incomplete, ambiguous, or irrelevant input can mislead diagnostic artificial intelligence tools. Therefore, rigorous refinement and verification processes are necessary to ensure data completeness and clarity, minimizing ambiguity and enhancing diagnostic reliability.

The evaluation of diagnostic performance typically involves either binary metrics or scale-based assessments. Binary metrics classify diagnostic outcomes as correct or incorrect. While this approach offers straightforward interpretation and ease of use, it inadequately addresses the subtleties of clinical diagnosis. For instance, a partially correct diagnosis may still offer substantial clinical utility, but binary metrics fail to acknowledge this complexity. For instance, an artificial intelligence that correctly identifies a patient has pneumonia but misidentifies the specific bacterial cause might be graded as "incorrect," yet its initial diagnosis still prompted life-saving antibiotic treatment, demonstrating significant clinical value. Particularly in standardized examinations and licensing tests, binary approaches dominate due to their simplicity, though they often overlook clinically significant nuances.

In contrast, scale-based assessments allow for more detailed evaluation by measuring diagnostic performance. For instance, the R-IDEA score, a validated 10-point scale, evaluates four core domains of clinical reasoning documentation: interpretive summary, differential diagnosis, explanation of lead diagnosis, and alternative diagnosis explained [4]. Such scales provide deeper insights and facilitate precise benchmarking against clinical standards. However, these scale-based assessments can introduce variability and subjective bias among evaluators. Differences in evaluators' interpretations and scoring approaches lead to inconsistencies, complicating comparisons across studies. Mitigating these challenges requires standardized evaluator training protocols coupled with objective metrics, enhancing both reliability and reproducibility of assessments.

Additionally, the appropriate number of differential diagnoses varies significantly based on clinical complexity and context. Simple cases often require fewer differentials, while complex scenarios necessitate more extensive lists [1]. Without predefined limits, artificial intelligence-driven tools may yield highly variable differential diagnoses, ranging from minimal to excessively extensive. Existing studies show variability from as few as 5 to as many as 40 differentials [5, 6]. Generative artificial intelligence systems, unlike traditional decision support systems, offer users the flexibility to explicitly define this number through tailored prompts, enhancing their utility in specific clinical or research contexts.

Finally, the translation of research findings into clinical practice faces significant hurdles, with a systematic review revealing that only 5% of studies evaluating artificial intelligence diagnostic performance utilize real patient data [7]. This highlights a critical gap in current evaluation methods, emphasizing the need for more practical and patient-centered validation studies. The iterative updating of artificial intelligence systems, leveraging continuous data integration, emerges as a vital strategy to refine and optimize their diagnostic performance. These ongoing refinements enable artificial intelligence tools to evolve, progressively enhancing their accuracy, reliability, and clinical relevance over time.

10.2.3 Limited Generalizability Across Populations

Another limitation arises from the generalizability of diagnostic systems. The prevalence of endemic diseases varies geographically. For instance, malaria is rarely included in the differential diagnosis for febrile patients in non-endemic areas without a travel history of international travel, whereas it is a routine consideration for febrile cases in endemic regions [8]. Diagnostic tools and algorithms trained on datasets specific to certain populations may fail to accommodate these regional variations. For example, a diagnostic system developed using data predominantly from non-endemic regions might overlook malaria entirely, leading to diagnostic errors. This highlights the need to train algorithms on datasets reflecting diverse geographic, demographic, and clinical realities. Including data from endemic and non-endemic regions during algorithm development can significantly improve the global applicability of these diagnostic tools. This limitation is particularly critical in global health contexts, where varying genetic, environmental, and lifestyle factors influence disease manifestation. Bridging this gap requires the inclusion of diverse and representative data during the development and validation phases. Beyond regional and population-specific challenges, diagnostic limitations also evolve over time as medical knowledge advances.

10.2.4 Temporal Limitations in Diagnosis

Medical knowledge and standards of care evolve over time, often rendering static diagnostic systems obsolete relatively quickly. For example, during ongoing pandemics caused by novel infectious diseases, scientific evidence is frequently updated daily [9]. This evidence often remains controversial until validated through high-quality and large-scale studies. Another example includes shifting terminology and understanding of diseases, such as the renaming of temporal arteritis to giant cell arteritis, which reflects updated medical consensus. This was because some patients did not display cranial symptoms or signs [10]. These dynamic changes emphasize the necessity for diagnostic systems to be continuously updated to remain aligned with current medical knowledge and standards. Artificial intelligence models trained on historical data may fail to account for recent advancements in medical science or changes in clinical guidelines. Moreover, there is often a time lag between the emergence of new findings and their incorporation into the learning datasets of artificial intelligence systems. Regular retraining of these systems with updated datasets is essential to bridge this gap and maintain their relevance and accuracy.

10.3 User-Related Limitations

Users of artificial intelligence in health care, including health-care professionals and patients, face unique challenges affecting diagnostic outcomes. Thorough awareness and understanding of these limitations are essential to mitigate associated risks and optimize the integration of artificial intelligence technologies in medical diagnostics.

10.3.1 Overreliance on Artificial Intelligence

Overreliance on artificial intelligence occurs when users uncritically accept artificial intelligence-generated recommendations, despite inaccuracies [11]. Excessive dependence on artificial intelligence systems can erode health-care professionals' critical thinking capabilities, increasing the risk of missing errors or anomalies not identified by artificial intelligence, thus potentially jeopardizing patient care and safety.

Health-care professionals and researchers frequently lack comprehensive artificial intelligence literacy, leading to new risks, including overreliance. Scientific literature has highlighted this phenomenon, especially following the rise of generative artificial intelligence platforms [12]. Studies reveal significant linguistic shifts in scientific writing [13, 14], with previously uncommon verbs such as "delve," and "showcase" dramatically increasing in usage within scientific outputs after the emergence of generative artificial intelligence. These features illustrate the influence of artificial intelligence-generated outputs on researcher behaviors, indicating potential erosion in critical thinking skills. Contributing factors include biased databases used for training artificial intelligence models, which inadequately capture diverse linguistic and disciplinary contexts, resulting in biased artificial intelligence outputs [15].

Although some linguistic trends are natural changes, the rapid pace and distinct pattern observed raise concerns about artificial intelligence's outsized influence on scientific communications [15]. Comprehensive research across various fields, languages, grammatical structures, and full manuscripts is necessary to validate these findings further. Similar influences could emerge in medical diagnostics as artificial intelligence systems become standard clinical tools. Therefore, continuous education and structured monitoring frameworks are vital to counteract artificial intelligence-induced biases and maintain robust critical assessment skills in health care.

10.3.2 Patient-Provided Information

Patients are integral to diagnostic accuracy through the information they provide. However, inadequate, inaccurate, or incomplete patient-provided information substantially elevates risks of misinformation and misdiagnosis. Commonly, patients omit essential details, often unaware of their significance, inadvertently supplying flawed diagnostic inputs.

The health-care community must emphasize educating patients about accurately and comprehensively conveying medical histories and symptoms. Documented cases illustrate that misuse or misunderstanding of generative artificial intelligence tools has resulted in diagnostic delays. In transient ischemic attacks, a case report revealed the need for patient education and effective patient-health care professional dialogue [16]. Strengthening this communication channel is essential to enhance artificial intelligence's diagnostic reliability.

10.3.3 "Black Box" Problem

The "black box" problem, referring to the inherent opacity of artificial intelligence algorithms, poses significant challenges to trust and interpretability in health-care settings [17]. Health-care professionals frequently face difficulties justifying artificial intelligence-informed decisions due to a lack of transparency, particularly in critical medical scenarios demanding clear rationales for clinical decisions. Consequently, patients and stakeholders find it challenging to trust and understand artificial intelligence-driven recommendations, diminishing the overall effectiveness and acceptance of artificial intelligence technologies.

To overcome this limitation, adopting and developing explainable artificial intelligence systems becomes crucial [18]. Explainable artificial intelligence enhances transparency, enabling health-care professionals to understand and communicate artificial intelligence-derived insights clearly and effectively to patients and stakeholders, ultimately fostering trust and acceptance. Addressing the "black box" problem comprehensively is critical, with detailed exploration provided in Sect. 6.2.2.

10.4 The Limitations Related to Artificial Intelligence

Artificial intelligence systems face challenges and limitations in their development and the environments in which they are applied.

10.4.1 Limitations in Artificial Intelligence Development

The impartiality of the artificial intelligence model is entirely dependent on the data used to train it. In medical diagnostics, biased datasets, whether due to underrepresentation of certain demographics or systemic inequities, can skew outcomes and perpetuate health disparities. Moreover, data quality and diversity remain pressing issues, as the complexity of medical data often requires extensive curation to ensure accuracy and representation. For example, large language models are typically developed using text data from the Internet. Consequently, due to the varying quality and quantity of this data, these systems often fail to perform effectively in diverse regional and cultural contexts [19, 20].

Additionally, artificial intelligence chatbots have emerged as valuable tools in health care by providing rapid and accessible medical information. However, disparities in several artificial intelligence chatbots for health-care responses are evident, depending on user location, platform, and the quality of training data [21]. These disparities raise concerns regarding health-care equity, accuracy, and accessibility, ultimately affecting patient outcomes. Understanding these variations is crucial to ensure that artificial intelligence-driven diagnostic tools deliver reliable and fair health-care information across different settings.

The absence of standardized data formats poses a significant challenge to integration, while inconsistent or incompatible datasets impede the seamless application of artificial intelligence across institutions and regions. For example, challenges such as data protection, patient privacy, and data security, as discussed in Chap. 11, further complicate the development process. Developing and deploying systems powered by artificial intelligence remains expensive. Computational resources, skilled personnel, and energy consumption, especially for large models such as those used in natural language processing, are cost-prohibitive for many institutions.

10.4.2 Environmental Limitation on the Adoption of Artificial Intelligence

Social acceptance and trust in systems based on artificial intelligence vary across different regions and communities. Factors such as mistrust, ethical concerns, and resistance to technological change considerably impede the widespread adoption of artificial intelligence technologies, especially in communities with limited exposure to advanced technologies. This societal dimension is critical, as it directly impacts the integration and practical effectiveness of artificial intelligence tools in medical diagnostics.

According to a global survey, the utilization of generative artificial intelligence tools among knowledge workers reaches approximately 75% worldwide, with substantial discrepancies observed across countries [22]. China exhibits a notably high adoption rate of 91%, driven largely by substantial national investment in artificial intelligence development and a supportive infrastructure designed for rapid technological growth. The United States shows a robust adoption rate of around 71%, which aligns with significant private sector initiatives, widespread digital literacy, and relatively flexible regulatory framework. In contrast, the United Kingdom (69%) and European Union countries such as Germany (69%), Spain (68%), and France (56%) show moderate adoption rates. This trend may result from stringent data regulations, including the General Data Protection Regulation. This regulation imposes stricter controls over data handling, privacy concerns, and ethical concerns with artificial intelligence. The European Union's careful approach towards balancing innovation with privacy and ethical considerations likely contributes to cautious adoption rates.

Japan represents a lower rate of artificial intelligence adoption, with only 32% of knowledge workers utilizing such tools. This can be attributed to a combination of cultural hesitation toward artificial intelligence-driven decision-making and a comparatively slower pace of digital transformation in some sectors, including health care [23].

In many low-resource settings, fundamental infrastructural limitations impede the deployment and effective use of artificial intelligence in medical diagnostics. Challenges such as unstable electricity supply and unreliable Internet connectivity can disrupt cloud-based artificial intelligence systems, undermining their reliability and performance [24]. These issues reinforce the digital divide, particularly disadvantaging regions that might benefit most from advanced diagnostic technologies. Bridging these infrastructural gaps is vital to ensuring equitable access to the benefits of artificial intelligence in health care globally.

10.4.3 Artificial Intelligence Maturity and Regulatory Standardization

The degree of artificial intelligence maturity within national health-care frameworks is another critical factor. According to the Broadband Commission for Sustainable Development, artificial intelligence maturity is categorized into three levels: Level 1 (Exploring), Level 2 (Emerging), and Level 3 (Integrated Ecosystem) [25]. Most Organization for Economic Cooperation and Development countries are currently at the Emerging stage, Level 2, indicating ongoing efforts to integrate artificial intelligence systems more deeply into health-care practice [26]. However, a lack of universal regulatory standards and guidelines complicates the progression to more advanced stages of artificial intelligence maturity. This absence of standardization not only impedes international research collaboration and data sharing but also creates inconsistencies in the development and application of artificial intelligence technologies across borders.

10.4.4 Political and Regulatory Hurdles

Political considerations and regulatory uncertainty further limit the widespread deployment of artificial intelligence in diagnostics. In some countries, restrictive policies or absence of clear regulations prevent the adoption of artificial intelligence tools, stifling innovation and access. International collaboration to establish universally accepted standards and guidelines is essential for overcoming these obstacles [27]. Such efforts can help ensure that the advantages of artificial intelligence technologies are equitably shared and that innovation in medical diagnostics is fostered on a global scale.

10.5 Other Limitations

Artificial intelligence in diagnostics is also limited by broader systemic and infrastructural challenges. These include ethical concerns regarding patient privacy and consent and challenges in integrating artificial intelligence into existing health care workflows. Ethical and legal considerations in artificial intelligence diagnostics are discussed in Chap. 11.

Integration with existing health care workflows also remains a critical challenge. Many health care systems rely on legacy software and processes that are incompatible with modern artificial intelligence platforms. This lack of compatibility can lead to inefficiencies, increased workload for health care professionals, and underutilization of artificial intelligence's capabilities. Addressing these issues requires coordinated efforts to modernize health care infrastructures and ensure seamless integration of artificial intelligence systems [28].

In summary, while artificial intelligence has potential in medical diagnostics, its limitations highlight the importance of careful and strategic implementation. Addressing the complexities of diagnosis itself, including challenges in defining, measuring, and generalizing diagnostic performance, is crucial for real-world applications. Overcoming these challenges requires cooperation among all stakeholders, including artificial intelligence developers, health-care professionals, policymakers, and society. Regularly updating datasets, refining systems for diverse populations, and incorporating new medical knowledge are essential to ensure that artificial intelligence remains a valuable tool in advancing health care.

References

1. Balogh EP, Miller BT, Ball JR. Improving diagnosis in health care. Washington, DC: National Academies Press; 2015.
2. Painter A, Hayhoe B, Riboli-Sasco E, El-Osta A. Online symptom checkers: recommendations for a vignette-based clinical evaluation standard. J Med Internet Res. 2022;24(10):e37408.
3. Liu Y, Cao J, Liu C, Ding K, Jin L. Datasets for large language models: A comprehensive survey. arXiv preprint arXiv:240218041. 2024.
4. Schaye V, Miller L, Kudlowitz D, Chun J, Burk-Rafel J, Cocks P, et al. Development of a clinical reasoning documentation assessment tool for resident and fellow admission notes: a shared mental model for feedback. J Gen Intern Med. 2022;37(3):507–12.
5. Berg HT, van Bakel B, van de Wouw L, Jie KE, Schipper A, Jansen H, et al. ChatGPT and generating a differential diagnosis early in an emergency department presentation. Ann Emerg Med. 2024;83(1):83–6.

6. Bridges JM. Computerized diagnostic decision support systems—a comparative performance study of Isabel Pro vs. ChatGPT4. Diagnosis Berl. 2024;11:250.
7. Bedi S, Liu Y, Orr-Ewing L, Dash D, Koyejo S, Callahan A, et al. Testing and evaluation of health care applications of large language models: a systematic review. JAMA. 2024;333(4):319–28.
8. Benelli G, Mehlhorn H. Declining malaria, rising of dengue and Zika virus: insights for mosquito vector control. Parasitol Res. 2016;115:1747–54.
9. Tabish SA. Covid-19 pandemic: emerging perspectives and future trends. J Public Health Res. 2020;9(1):jphr.2020.1786.
10. Gonzalez-Gay MA, Garcia-Porrua C, Amor-Dorado JC, Llorca J. Giant cell arteritis without clinically evident vascular involvement in a defined population. Arthritis Care Res. 2004;51(2):274–7.
11. Passi S, Vorvoreanu M. Overreliance on AI Literature Review. 2022. Available from: https://www.microsoft.com/en-us/research/uploads/prod/2022/06/Aether-Overreliance-on-AI-Review-Final-6.21.22.pdf
12. Teh PL, Uwasomba CF. Impact of large language models on scholarly publication titles and abstracts: a comparative analysis. J Soc Comput. 2024;5(2):105–21.
13. Geng M, Trotta R. Human-LLM Coevolution: Evidence from Academic Writing. arXiv preprint arXiv:250209606. 2025.
14. Liang W, Izzo Z, Zhang Y, Lepp H, Cao H, Zhao X, et al. Monitoring AI-modified content at scale: a case study on the impact of ChatGPT on AI conference peer reviews. arXiv preprint arXiv:240307183. 2024.
15. Dergaa I, Chamari K, Zmijewski P, Saad HB. From human writing to artificial intelligence generated text: examining the prospects and potential threats of ChatGPT in academic writing. Biol Sport. 2023;40(2):615–22.
16. Saenger JA, Hunger J, Boss A, Richter J. Delayed diagnosis of a transient ischemic attack caused by ChatGPT. Wien Klin Wochenschr. 2024;136(7–8):236–8.
17. Ashok M, Madan R, Joha A, Sivarajah U. Ethical framework for artificial intelligence and digital technologies. Int J Inf Manag. 2022;62:102433.
18. Angelov PP, Soares EA, Jiang R, Arnold NI, Atkinson PM. Explainable artificial intelligence: an analytical review. WIREs Data Min Knowl Discov. 2021;11(5):e1424.
19. Wach K, Duong CD, Ejdys J, Kazlauskaitė R, Korzynski P, Mazurek G, et al. The dark side of generative artificial intelligence: a critical analysis of controversies and risks of ChatGPT. Entrep Bus Econ Rev. 2023;11(2):7–30.
20. Choudhury M. Generative AI has a language problem. Nat Hum Behav. 2023;7(11):1802–3.
21. Gumilar KE, Indraprasta BR, Hsu Y-C, Yu Z-Y, Chen H, Irawan B, et al. Disparities in medical recommendations from AI-based chatbots across different countries/regions. Sci Rep. 2024;14(1):17052.
22. Microsoft, LinkedIn. 2024 Work Trend Index Annual Report Microsoft; 2024. Available from: https://www.microsoft.com/en-us/worklab/work-trend-index/ai-at-work-is-here-now-comes-the-hard-part
23. Dwivedi YK, Hughes L, Ismagilova E, Aarts G, Coombs C, Crick T, et al. Artificial intelligence (AI): multidisciplinary perspectives on emerging challenges, opportunities, and agenda for research, practice and policy. Int J Inf Manag. 2021;57:101994.
24. Dangi RR, Sharma A, Vageriya V. Transforming healthcare in low-resource settings with artificial intelligence: recent developments and outcomes. Public Health Nurs. 2025;42(2):1017–30.
25. Commission B. Reimagining Global Health through Artificial Intelligence: The Roadmap to AI Maturity 2020. Available from: https://broadbandcommission.org/wp-content/uploads/2021/02/WGAIinHealth_Report2020.pdf
26. Castonguay A, Wagner G, Motulsky A, Paré G. AI maturity in health care: an overview of 10 OECD countries. Health Policy. 2024;140:104938.
27. Taeihagh A. Governance of artificial intelligence. Polic Soc. 2021;40(2):137–57.
28. Gopal G, Suter-Crazzolara C, Toldo L, Eberhardt W. Digital transformation in healthcare—architectures of present and future information technologies. Clin Chem Lab Med. 2019;57(3):328–35.

Ethical and Regulatory Considerations in AI Diagnostics

11

Abstract

This chapter addresses the ethical and regulatory challenges for artificial intelligence in medical diagnostics. Key ethical considerations include explainability, balancing transparency with accuracy, and ensuring human autonomy amid increasing automation. This chapter highlights issues like bias, fairness, and the risks posed by generative artificial intelligence tools. Regulatory frameworks, such as the Health Insurance Portability and Accountability Act in the United States and the General Data Protection Regulation in the European Union, are analyzed for their roles in safeguarding data privacy, security, and transparency. Their limitations in keeping pace with artificial intelligence advancements are acknowledged. The chapter emphasizes the need for global, adaptive standards to ensure ethical and effective artificial intelligence implementation in health care.

Keywords

Explainability · Interpretability · Fidelity · Autonomy · Human Oversight · Bias · Transparency · Privacy

11.1 Ethical Considerations in AI Diagnostics

The use of artificial intelligence in health care, especially in medical diagnostics, presents significant ethical challenges. All stakeholders interacting with artificial intelligence, including health-care professionals, developers, regulatory officials, policymakers, patients, and their families, all play important roles in ensuring the ethical development, improvement, and implementation of artificial intelligence systems.

T. Hirosawa, *Artificial Intelligence in Medical Diagnostics*,
https://doi.org/10.1007/978-981-95-4338-0_11

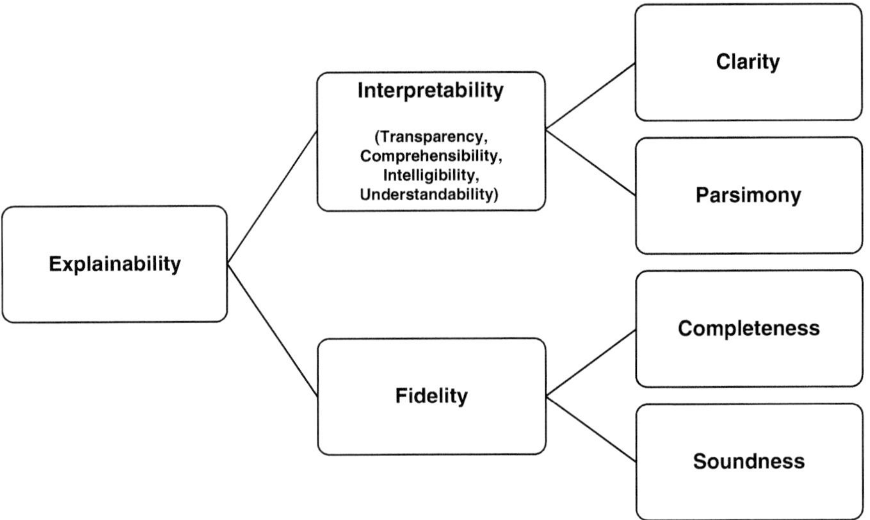

Fig. 11.1 Components of explainability, showing interpretability (clarity, parsimony) and fidelity (completeness, soundness)

11.1.1 Explainability

One of the most critical aspects of ethical artificial intelligence is explainability, the ability to make artificial intelligence decisions interpretable and understandable for all stakeholders. Some researchers do not specify what terms mean, often using the same term for different meanings or referring to the same concept with different terminology. Explainability in artificial intelligence diagnostics refers to the extent to which the decisions made by an artificial intelligence system can be understood, justified, and trusted by its users, including health-care professionals and patients. Explainability addresses two critical questions [1]:

1. Why did the artificial intelligence system make a particular decision? (Interpretability).
2. How reliable or accurate is artificial intelligence's explanation? (Fidelity).

Figure 11.1 summarizes the key components of explainability, including interpretability and fidelity, and highlights associated attributes like clarity, parsimony, completeness, and soundness [2].

11.1.2 Interpretability

Interpretability refers to the degree to which the internal workings of an artificial intelligence system can be understood by human users. An interpretable artificial intelligence system provides insights into how it processes inputs to generate outputs. It includes terms as follows:

- Transparency: The ability to observe and understand how an artificial intelligence system operates. For instance, in a rule-based diagnostic CDSS, a health-care professional can see and comprehend each step the model took to arrive at a diagnosis.
- Comprehensibility: How easily a human can grasp the logic behind artificial intelligence decisions. For example, a simple decision tree used to predict disease outcomes is more comprehensible than a deep neural network [3].
- Intelligibility and Understandability: The clarity of artificial intelligence explanation. An artificial intelligence predicting the likelihood of heart disease should present its reasoning in clear, plain language, such as explaining how cholesterol levels, blood pressure, and age contributed to the prediction.

Interpretability is further supported by the attributes of the following:

- Clarity: Explanations must be unambiguous and understandable to nonexpert users. For instance, artificial intelligence's output presented as "low risk" or "high risk" is clearer than complex clinical prediction scores.
- Parsimony: Parsimony emphasizes simplicity in explanation, avoiding unnecessary complexity. For example, providing concise step-by-step reasoning for diagnosing pneumonia based on radiographic features ensures that health-care professionals can quickly interpret the artificial intelligence's decision.

11.1.3 Fidelity

Fidelity measures how accurately an explanation aligns with the actual functioning of the artificial intelligence system. An explanation is faithful if it truthfully represents the model's decision-making process. Even if a system appears interpretable, its explanations are meaningless unless they accurately reflect the underlying reasoning process. Fidelity ensures that the explanation:

- Represents the true logic behind the model's decision, rather than creating superficial or misleading reasoning.
- Does not oversimplify complex relationships at the cost of accuracy.

Fidelity is closely related to the following:

- Completeness: The explanation should provide a comprehensive understanding of the decision. For example, in an artificial intelligence system for medical imaging, explanations must include all critical features the artificial intelligence considered, such as lung opacities or nodular shadows, rather than presenting partial reasoning. It is worth noting that some researchers used the term "completeness" interchangeably with "fidelity" [4].
- Soundness: Soundness ensures that the explanation aligns with clinical standards and logical reasoning. For instance, artificial intelligence diagnosing diabetes

mellitus should justify its prediction based on medically accepted thresholds for fasting blood glucose or HbA1c levels.

11.1.4 Balancing Explainability and Accuracy

Explainability is a cornerstone of ethical artificial intelligence in diagnostics, ensuring that artificial intelligence systems are transparent, interpretable, and trustworthy. However, there is often a trade-off between explainability and accuracy [5]. Complex models, such as artificial neural networks, may achieve higher predictive accuracy but at the expense of reduced interpretability. For instance, a highly accurate deep learning model might correctly predict a patient's risk of sepsis with 95% accuracy but be unable to explain why, whereas a simpler, less accurate decision tree model might only be 85% accurate but can show the exact clinical factors (e.g., "high white blood cell count AND low blood pressure") that led to its conclusion. Artificial neural networks are discussed in Chap. 4.

Addressing this trade-off requires careful design by artificial intelligence developers. By incorporating components such as interpretability, fidelity, completeness, and soundness into the design process, artificial intelligence systems can better align with clinical needs and ethical standards. Developers should strive for solutions that maximize both accuracy and explainability, fostering trust and usability among diverse stakeholders in medical diagnostics.

11.1.5 Automation and Human Autonomy

Automation refers to the process by which systems or machines perform tasks with reduced human intervention. Autonomy, on the other hand, denotes the ability of a system to make decisions and operate independently. Together, these concepts define how responsibilities are shared between humans and machines in various contexts, including health care. There are various levels of automation. While Sheridan defined 10 levels using a "who-centered" approach, Endsley and Kaber defined another 10 levels using an information-sharing and situation awareness perspective. Endsley later expanded the levels to 12 [6].

In Table 11.1, Endsley's levels range from manual control, Level 1, where humans perform all tasks, to full automation, Level 12, where the computer performs all tasks without human intervention. Intermediate levels describe increasing computer assistance, including cueing information (Level 2), shared decision-making (Level 6), blended decision-making with human consent (Level 8), and supervisory control (Level 11). Sheridan's levels emphasize task division, where the human transitions from complete control, Level 1, to limited oversight while the system selects, implements, and even explains actions, Levels 8–10 [6].

Endsley and Kiris define five levels of automation, starting with no system involvement. At the lowest level, humans decide and act independently. Decision support involves artificial intelligence suggesting actions while humans decide and

Table 11.1 Endsley's 12 levels of automation [6]

Level	Label	Definition
1	Manual control	The human is responsible for performing all aspects of the task
2	Information cueing	Prompts or highlights critical data to aid decision-making
3	Situation awareness support	System gathers and integrates information to enhance user awareness, particularly for levels 2 and 3 processes
4	Action support/ teleoperation	System follows instructions to carry out specific actions as directed by the human operator
5	Batch processing	System independently completes single or multiple tasks once commanded by the human
6	Shared control	Human and system generate possible choices together; human makes the final decision and executes it with system support
7	Decision support	System generates options, human chooses or inputs their own, and system executes the action
8	Blended decision-making	System proposes options and a preferred choice, but execution requires explicit human approval (or supervision)
9	Constrained choice	System presents a fixed set of options from which the human must select, after which the system carries out the action
10	Automated decision-making	Both human and system generate alternatives; system selects the best and performs, with human in a secondary role
11	Supervisory control	System selects and executes the best option but allows human intervention if necessary (management by exception)
12	Full automation	System performs all aspects of the task without any human involvement

act. At consensual artificial intelligence levels, both the artificial intelligence and human must agree before actions occur. Monitored artificial intelligence allows the system to act but gives humans veto power. Full automation is the highest level, where the artificial intelligence acts independently without human input [7].

From these contexts, artificial intelligence system autonomy can be categorized into five levels. Level 0 represents standard care with no artificial intelligence involvement, where humans make all decisions. Level 1 involves artificial intelligence assisting by suggesting decisions, but humans retain control. In Level 2, artificial intelligence makes decisions under human supervision. At Level 3, artificial intelligence acts independently but notifies humans when necessary. Finally, Level 4 involves fully autonomous artificial intelligence that operates without human backup, including decision-making, as depicted in Table 11.2 [8].

All these frameworks describe progression from human control to full automation. They emphasize the gradual transition of responsibility from humans to systems, ranging from supportive roles to shared control, supervisory roles, and, finally, complete autonomy. While these frameworks differ slightly, they converge on critical themes of trust, oversight, and accountability as automation increases.

In the context of automation and artificial intelligence, human autonomy refers to the capacity of individuals to make independent decisions, exercise control, and maintain agency in environments increasingly influenced by automated systems. As automation levels increase, preserving human autonomy becomes critical to ensure trust, ethical oversight, and effective collaboration between humans and artificial intelligence systems. Balancing the capabilities of autonomous systems with the

Table 11.2 Artificial intelligence (AI) system autonomy level [7, 8]

AI system autonomy Levels	Definition	Final decision	Endsley & Kiris (1995)
Level 0	No AI	Human	None
Level 1	AI suggests decisions to human	Human	Decision support
Level 2	AI makes decisions with human supervision	Human	Consensual AI
Level 3	AI makes decisions with no continuous supervision	AI	Monitored AI
Level 4	Full AI autonomy (no human backup)	AI	Full automation

need for meaningful human involvement requires careful consideration of factors such as decision-making thresholds, the role of human oversight, and the potential consequences of overreliance on automation. This ensures that humans remain active participants, especially in high-stakes domains such as health care, where the nuances of human judgment and ethical reasoning are indispensable [9].

11.1.6 Ethical Considerations for Generative Artificial Intelligence

With the introduction of generative artificial intelligence, large language models have received enormous attention in health care [10, 11]. Despite their potential benefits, researchers have emphasized various ethical implications. A review article identifies recurring ethical concerns. One significant concern is fairness and bias, which refers to the potential for perpetuating existing biases in health-care datasets. Non-maleficence emerges as another critical issue, highlighting the risks of producing harmful or misleading content [12]. Transparency presents challenges in understanding how large language models generate their outputs, while privacy highlights the importance of protecting sensitive patient data. A distinctive concern is the tendency of large language models to produce harmful or convincing but inaccurate content. Calls for ethical guidance and human oversight are recurrent [13]. Beyond ethical concerns, the rapid adoption of artificial intelligence in diagnostics also raises critical regulatory questions.

11.2 Regulatory Considerations in Artificial Intelligence

The rapid advancement of artificial intelligence, particularly in health care and diagnostics, has introduced significant challenges for existing regulatory frameworks. Regulations aim to safeguard patient privacy, data security, and ethical use while fostering innovation [14]. Over 100 countries have enacted data protection laws to address privacy and data security [15]. Some guidelines, such as the Ibero-American Data Protection Network, are designed specifically to manage the use of personal data for artificial intelligence [16]. However, the rapid evolution of artificial intelligence technologies often outpaces the development of comprehensive legal and regulatory frameworks. Two major regulatory frameworks influencing artificial intelligence in diagnostics are Health Insurance Portability and Accountability Act (HIPAA) in the United States and General Data Protection Regulation (GDPR) in the European Union.

11.2.1 Health Insurance Portability and Accountability Act

HIPAA is the primary regulation in the United States governing the privacy and security of patients' health information. Enacted in 1996, HIPAA was designed to ensure that patients' medical data remains confidential while allowing for appropriate sharing of information for treatment, payment, and health-care operations [17].

In the realm of artificial intelligence-based medical tools and diagnostics, HIPAA imposes several critical requirements that directly shape system design, development, and deployment:

- Protected Health Information: Artificial intelligence systems processing patient data for diagnostics must comply with HIPAA regulations to protect health information, such as names, medical record numbers, and imaging data. For instance, an artificial intelligence tool analyzing computed tomography scans must ensure that the associated patient metadata is anonymized and securely stored.
- Data Privacy and Security: HIPAA requires artificial intelligence developers and health-care providers to implement robust safeguards, such as encryption, access controls, and secure storage protocols. Artificial intelligence systems must prevent unauthorized access to sensitive data during training, deployment, and inference phases.
- Third-Party Artificial Intelligence Vendors: If health-care organizations use artificial intelligence tools developed by third-party vendors, those vendors must sign Business Associate Agreements to confirm their compliance with HIPAA standards.

Despite HIPAA's importance, applying its provisions to the dynamic, data-intensive world of artificial intelligence diagnostics presents several challenges:

- De-Identification: Artificial intelligence systems often require vast amounts of data for training. While HIPAA permits the use of de-identified data without patient consent, achieving true de-identification—such as removing identifying details from genomic and genetic data—can be challenging and prone to re-identification risks [18].
- Data Sharing and Cross-Institution Collaboration: HIPAA creates challenges for data sharing across institutions, as its framework was not designed to govern the large-scale, multi-organizational "big data" projects common in artificial intelligence development. Furthermore, HIPAA's jurisdiction is generally limited to health-care organizations and does not cover the vast health-related datasets

handled by technology giant companies, which further complicates the regulatory landscape [19]. Striking a balance between innovation and compliance in this environment requires significant effort.

11.2.2 General Data Protection Regulation (GDPR)

The GDPR is the European Union's data protection framework, enacted in 2018, which governs the collection, processing, and storage of personal data, including health data. Unlike HIPAA, which is specific to the health-care sector, GDPR applies broadly to all data types and industries, including artificial intelligence-driven health-care systems [20]. Its overarching purpose is to protect the fundamental freedoms and rights of individuals, particularly regarding how their personal data is controlled and processed by third parties [21].

The GDPR imposes concrete responsibilities on developers, hospitals, and technology providers:

- Data Minimization: Artificial intelligence systems must collect only the data necessary for their intended purpose. For example, an artificial intelligence tool designed to predict lung cancer from X-rays should avoid collecting unrelated data.
- Lawfulness, Fairness, and Transparency: Patients must provide explicit consent for the use of their data. Artificial intelligence developers must clearly explain how patient data will be processed, ensuring transparency.
- Right to Explanation: GDPR includes provisions for the "right to explanation," requiring organizations to provide clear justifications for automated decisions made by artificial intelligence systems. This aligns with ethical principles of explainability (see Sect. 11.1).
- Data Portability and Erasure (Right to Be Forgotten): Patients can request their data to be transferred or deleted. Artificial intelligence developers must design systems capable of identifying and removing specific patient data when requested.

While GDPR provides a robust framework for protecting individuals, its application in artificial intelligence-based diagnostics poses significant challenges:

- Informed Consent: Obtaining valid and explicit consent for the use of data in artificial intelligence systems can be challenging, particularly for preventing opt-out based participation [20].
- Artificial Intelligence Interpretability and the Right to Explanation: Complex artificial intelligence models, such as deep learning, often function as "black boxes" [22]. Meeting the GDPR requirement necessitates that developers ensure artificial intelligence decisions are interpretable and understandable to users.
- Cross-Border Data Transfer: GDPR imposes strict regulations on transferring personal data outside the European Union, which can hinder international collaborations for artificial intelligence development in diagnostics [23].

11.2.3 Speed of Artificial Intelligence Development Versus Regulatory Frameworks

Despite the efforts of HIPAA and GDPR to regulate data privacy and security, legal frameworks often fail to keep pace with the rapid development of artificial intelligence in health care [8, 24]. Representative areas where regulation lags include the following:

- Evolving Artificial Intelligence Capabilities: State-of-the-art artificial intelligence can identify patterns in complex datasets, such as radiology images or genomic data, with unprecedented accuracy [25, 26]. However, regulators struggle to define standards for validating artificial intelligence algorithms, ensuring fairness, and monitoring bias.
- Global Disparities in Regulation: While HIPAA and GDPR provide strong precedents, many countries lack equivalent frameworks. This creates inconsistencies in data governance and patient protection, particularly for artificial intelligence tools deployed internationally [27].
- Ethical and Accountability Challenges: Regulatory frameworks often focus on data privacy but lack clear guidelines for ethical considerations like fairness, bias mitigation, and accountability [28]. For example, who is legally responsible when an artificial intelligence system leads to diagnostic error—developers, health-care professionals, or the institution?
- Quick Adaptation of Artificial Intelligence Systems: Many artificial intelligence models are dynamic, meaning they continue to learn and adapt as new data becomes available. Regulatory processes, which typically involve static evaluations, struggle to keep up with these evolving systems.
- Artificial Intelligence Bias and Fairness: Regulations currently lack explicit standards for detecting and mitigating bias in artificial intelligence. As discussed in Sect. 1.2.3, biased training datasets can result in artificial intelligence models that perform poorly for underrepresented groups, exacerbating health-care disparities [29].

HIPAA, GDPR, and other guidelines represent essential regulatory frameworks for ensuring privacy, security, and ethical data use in artificial intelligence diagnostics. However, these regulations were not originally designed for the complexities introduced by modern artificial intelligence. As artificial intelligence technologies continue to evolve, regulatory bodies must adapt quickly to address emerging challenges such as transparency, fairness, and accountability. Current regulatory shifts, such as efforts to classify certain digital health-care applications as medical devices, also open the door to systematic reporting and oversight of artificial intelligence-related incidents, signaling a move toward more proactive governance [30]. Policymakers must work alongside technologists, health-care providers, and ethicists to establish agile, global standards that foster innovation while protecting patient rights and safety.

In summary, the integration of artificial intelligence into medical diagnostics offers transformative opportunities but also raises significant ethical and regulatory challenges. This chapter highlighted the importance of explainability, involving interpretability and fidelity, as essential for building trust and usability among stakeholders. Balancing explainability and accuracy, addressing bias, and ensuring ethical automation remain critical for aligning artificial intelligence systems with clinical needs and ethical principles. Regulatory frameworks like HIPAA and GDPR provide a foundation for data privacy and security but struggle to keep pace with rapid artificial intelligence advancements. Bridging this gap requires adaptive policies, global collaboration, and robust standards to safeguard patient rights while fostering innovation. The next chapter introduces interdisciplinary collaboration, emphasizing how partnerships among health-care professionals, computer scientists, ethicists, and policymakers play a pivotal role in translating artificial intelligence from research into safe, equitable, and effective applications across medical diagnostics and other professional domains.

References

1. Afroogh S, Akbari A, Malone E, Kargar M, Alambeigi H. Trust in AI: progress, challenges, and future directions. Human So Sci Commun. 2024;11(1):1568.
2. Markus AF, Kors JA, Rijnbeek PR. The role of explainability in creating trustworthy artificial intelligence for health care: a comprehensive survey of the terminology, design choices, and evaluation strategies. J Biomed Inform. 2021;113:103655.
3. Sakr S, Elshawi R, Ahmed AM, Qureshi WT, Brawner CA, Keteyian SJ, et al. Comparison of machine learning techniques to predict all-cause mortality using fitness data: the Henry ford exercIse testing (FIT) project. BMC Med Inform Decis Mak. 2017;17(1):174.
4. Gilpin LH, Bau D, Yuan BZ, Bajwa A, Specter M, Kagal L, editors. Explaining explanations: an overview of interpretability of machine learning. 2018 IEEE 5th international conference on data science and advanced analytics (DSAA); 2018 1–3 Oct 2018.
5. London AJ. Artificial intelligence and black-box medical decisions: accuracy versus explainability. Hastings Cent Rep. 2019;49(1):15–21.
6. Abbass HA. Social integration of artificial intelligence: functions, automation allocation logic and human-autonomy trust. Cogn Comput. 2019;11(2):159–71.
7. Endsley MR. Automation and situation awareness. In: Automation and human performance. CRC Press; 2018. p. 163–81.
8. Mennella C, Maniscalco U, De Pietro G, Esposito M. Ethical and regulatory challenges of AI technologies in healthcare: a narrative review. Heliyon. 2024;10(4):e26297.
9. Karimian G, Petelos E, Evers SM. The ethical issues of the application of artificial intelligence in healthcare: a systematic scoping review. AI Ethics 2022;2(4):539–551.
10. Javaid M, Haleem A, Singh RP. ChatGPT for healthcare services: an emerging stage for an innovative perspective. BenchCouncil Trans Benchmarks Standards Evaluat. 2023;3(1):100105.
11. Liu J, Wang C, Liu S. Utility of ChatGPT in clinical practice. J Med Internet Res. 2023;25:e48568.
12. Tang L, Sun Z, Idnay B, Nestor JG, Soroush A, Elias PA, et al. Evaluating large language models on medical evidence summarization. NPJ Digit Med. 2023;6(1):158.
13. Haltaufderheide J, Ranisch R. The ethics of ChatGPT in medicine and healthcare: a systematic review on large language models (LLMs). NPJ Digit Med. 2024;7(1):183.
14. Kanter GP, Packel EA. Health care privacy risks of AI chatbots. JAMA. 2023;330(4):311–2.
15. WHO. Ethics and governance of artificial intelligence for health: WHO guidance. 2021.
16. de RIdP, Datos. Specific guidelines for compliance with the principles and rights that govern the protection of personal data in artificial intelligence projects Brussels: European Union; 2019. Available from: https://www.redipd.org/en/documents/guide-specific-guidelines-ai-projects

17. Act A. Health insurance portability and accountability act of 1996. Public law 1996;104:191.
18. Kulynych J, Greely HT. Clinical genomics, big data, and electronic medical records: reconciling patient rights with research when privacy and science collide. J Law Biosci. 2017;4(1):94–132.
19. Price WN 2nd, Cohen IG. Privacy in the age of medical big data. Nat Med. 2019;25(1):37–43.
20. Forcier MB, Gallois H, Mullan S, Joly Y. Integrating artificial intelligence into health care through data access: can the GDPR act as a beacon for policymakers? J Law Biosci. 2019;6(1):317–35.
21. Room S. Data protection and compliance in context. Swindon: British Computer Society; 2007.
22. Von Eschenbach WJ. Transparency and the black box problem: why we do not trust AI. Philos Technol. 2021;34(4):1607–22.
23. Draghi M. The future of European competitiveness part B: in-depth analysis and recommendations. 2024.
24. Taeihagh A. Governance of artificial intelligence. Polic Soc. 2021;40(2):137–57.
25. Kelly BS, Judge C, Bollard SM, Clifford SM, Healy GM, Aziz A, et al. Radiology artificial intelligence: a systematic review and evaluation of methods (RAISE). Eur Radiol. 2022;32(11):7998–8007.
26. Quazi S. Artificial intelligence and machine learning in precision and genomic medicine. Med Oncol. 2022;39(8):120.
27. Cihon P, Maas MM, Kemp L. Fragmentation and the future: investigating architectures for international AI governance. Global Pol. 2020;11(5):545–56.
28. Zhou N, Zhang Z, Nair VN, Singhal H, Chen J. Bias, fairness and accountability with artificial intelligence and machine learning algorithms. Int Stat Rev. 2022;90(3):468–80.
29. Challen R, Denny J, Pitt M, Gompels L, Edwards T, Tsaneva-Atanasova K. Artificial intelligence, bias and clinical safety. BMJ Qual Saf. 2019;28(3):231–7.
30. Pruski M. AI-enhanced healthcare: not a new paradigm for informed consent. J Bioethical Inquiry. 2024;21(3):475–89.

Interdisciplinary Collaboration for AI Development

12

Abstract

Interdisciplinary collaboration plays a pivotal role in developing and applying artificial intelligence across various professional domains, including medical diagnostics. Integrating diverse expertise enables researchers, developers, and professionals to tackle complex challenges, optimize workflows, and produce transformative solutions. Specifically, artificial intelligence-driven medical diagnostics benefit from collaborations involving health-care professionals, data scientists, engineers, and ethicists. This chapter discusses successful case studies from multiple disciplines, demonstrating the profound impact interdisciplinary collaboration can have on artificial intelligence-enhanced performance and groundbreaking achievements.

Keywords

Collaboration · Board Game · Sports analytics · Predictive analytics · Ethical considerations · Human–AI partnership

12.1 Interdisciplinary Collaboration in Health Care and Beyond

Interdisciplinary collaboration is central to advancing artificial intelligence in health care, combining diverse expertise to solve complex challenges. Such collaborations occur on various levels, including cross-specialty medical teams, specialists-generalists' interactions, and partnerships with patients. Each level of collaboration enriches diagnostic precision and therapeutic effectiveness by integrating distinct perspectives and specialized knowledge.

T. Hirosawa, *Artificial Intelligence in Medical Diagnostics*,
https://doi.org/10.1007/978-981-95-4338-0_12

12.1.1 Collaboration among Health-Care Professionals

Effective interdisciplinary collaboration among health-care professionals fosters a comprehensive approach to patient care. Specialists from different disciplines bring unique insights, enabling solutions to complex problems that single-domain expertise might not resolve [1]. Furthermore, interactions between specialists and generalists are crucial for comprehensive diagnostics, as they merge highly specialized knowledge with broader patient-centered perspectives. Chapter 7 highlights collective diagnosis, emphasizing the critical role of diverse expert collaboration in enhancing clinical decision-making accuracy.

12.1.2 Collaboration Between Health-Care Professionals and Patients

Collaboration between health-care professionals and patients is integral to developing patient-centered artificial intelligence solutions. Engaging patients in artificial intelligence tool development ensures technologies address actual patient needs, remain user-friendly, and enhance accessibility across diverse populations. Studies reveal patients harbor concerns about artificial intelligence-related safety, autonomy, health-care cost implications, data biases, and data security [2]. Addressing these concerns transparently and ethically is essential to cultivating patient trust, which is critical for widespread adoption and success of artificial intelligence applications in health care.

12.1.3 Collaboration Between Health-Care Professionals and Artificial Intelligence Developers

Close collaboration between health-care professionals and artificial intelligence developers is pivotal for aligning technological innovation with clinical realities. Health-care professionals provide essential clinical insights, guiding artificial intelligence developers in algorithm refinement, data validation, and ethical compliance. Such partnerships ensure artificial intelligence solutions are practical, effective, and ethically aligned, ultimately enhancing patient outcomes and ensuring safety in real-world settings.

12.1.4 Collaboration Between Health-Care Professionals and Other Experts

Beyond health care and artificial intelligence development, interdisciplinary collaborations include experts from diverse, non-medical fields such as engineering, bioinformatics, psychology, sociology, law, and ethics. These experts significantly contribute to creating artificial intelligence solutions that are technologically innovative, ethically robust, and human-centric.

Psychologists play a crucial role in designing intuitive user interfaces for artificial intelligence applications, ensuring ease of use and effective interactions for both medical staff and patients [3]. Sociologists analyze artificial intelligence's societal implications, focusing on equity, health-care accessibility, and public perceptions, thus informing socially responsible artificial intelligence development [4]. Legal professionals and ethicists help health-care professionals navigate complex regulatory landscapes and ethical dilemmas, ensuring compliance and promoting responsible artificial intelligence adoption [5]. Collectively, these interdisciplinary efforts ensure that artificial intelligence advancements in medical diagnostics are both technologically sound and socially responsible, ultimately benefiting broader health-care ecosystems and societal welfare.

12.2 Case Studies for Interdisciplinary Collaboration

By examining case studies from diverse sectors, we gain valuable insights into the mechanisms of interdisciplinary collaboration involving artificial intelligence. Such case studies illuminate how experts across various fields successfully collaborate with artificial intelligence systems to tackle challenges, redefine traditional methodologies, and unlock new possibilities. Central to these examples is the recognition of openness, mutual respect among professionals, and strategic integration of artificial intelligence to enhance outcomes and drive innovation. A summary highlighting key lessons from interdisciplinary collaboration involving artificial intelligence developments is presented in Table 12.1.

12.2.1 Shogi

Shogi, commonly known as "Japanese chess," represents a compelling instance of interdisciplinary collaboration, involving professional Shogi players and artificial intelligence researchers. Although Shogi shares basic principles with Western chess, including piece movement and the objective of checkmating an opponent's king, Shogi introduces unique complexities. The key difference is the ability to reintroduce captured pieces back into play, significantly increasing the strategic depth and computational demands of the game [6].

As shown in Table 12.2, a comparison of Shogi and chess across five key categories—board size, number of pieces, number of different types of pieces, game-tree complexity, and average game length—highlights their differences. Shogi has a 9×9 board, 40 pieces, 8 different types of pieces, and an average game length of 110 moves. In contrast, chess is played on an 8×8 board with 32 pieces, 6 different types of pieces, and an average game length of 80 moves [7]. The computational demands of Shogi far exceed those of chess: while the state-space complexity of chess is approximately 10^{43}, that of Shogi is estimated at 10^{71}. Similarly, the game-tree complexity of chess is around 10^{123}, whereas for Shogi it is an astronomical 10^{226} [8]. These magnitudes illustrate the immense challenge posed to artificial

Table 12.1 Summary of interdisciplinary collaboration for artificial intelligence (AI) developments in medical diagnostics, shogi, baseball, and football

Aspect	Medical diagnostics	Shogi	Baseball	Football
Domain characteristics	Complex, dynamic variables in patient data, comorbidities, and diverse clinical contexts	Highly structured rules, dynamic strategies, large branching factor	Structured environment with measurable player and game data	Dynamic, multiagent environment with continuous movement and interactions
Role of AI	Enhances diagnostic accuracy via dataset analysis and disease prediction	Suggests novel strategies through unbiased game-state analysis	Optimizes performance, predicts outcomes, prevents injuries via analytics	Analyzes performance, optimizes team strategy, predicts injury risks
Type of collaboration	Collaboration among health care professionals, data scientists, ethicists, and policymakers	Collaboration between professional players and AI developers	Collaboration among players, coaches, sports scientists, and AI engineers	Collaboration among coaches, players, medical staff, sports scientists, and data analysts
Key challenges	Data privacy, ethical concerns, health care professional trust, patient safety	High computational complexity from branching factors	Integrating AI with human decision-making, ensuring player compliance	Integrating real-time data from multiple sources, managing player adoption
Lessons for AI adoption	Adaptive, context-aware systems validated across populations	Iterative learning and unbiased evaluation for strategy refinement	Predictive analytics and feedback loops for continuous improvement	Predictive analytics and real-time feedback for performance and safety
Differences in impact	Impact on patient health and safety, requiring strict validation and ethics	Influence limited to game strategies without long-term external impact	Impact on game results and team performance, reversible in future matches	Impact on outcomes and careers, adaptable in subsequent matches

Table 12.2 Representative characteristics between shogi and chess

Game	Shogi	Chess
Popular region	Japan	Europe
Basic characteristics		
Board size	9×9	8×8
Number of pieces	40	32
Types of pieces	8	6
Average moves per game	110	80
Computational demands		
State-space complexity	10^{71}	10^{43}
Game-tree complexity	10^{226}	10^{123}

intelligence systems, as the larger board and exponential growth in potential move sequences dramatically increase the complexity of analysis and decision-making.

An exemplary case of interdisciplinary success is observed in the career of Sota Fuji, a prodigious young player renowned for breaking historic records [9]. Fuji's integration of artificial intelligence tools into his practice facilitated his exploration of unconventional strategies that might typically be overlooked by human players. Reflecting on this, Fuji stated, "We humans are likely to dismiss certain ideas, based on our experiences or preconceptions, but artificial intelligence considers all of them" [10].

This highlights the capacity of artificial intelligence algorithms—particularly those employing deep reinforcement learning and Monte Carlo Tree Search—to provide unbiased assessments of vast potential moves, thereby augmenting human decision-making [11]. Deep reinforcement learning involves artificial intelligence agents learning optimal moves through environmental interactions, guided by rewards or penalties, while Monte Carlo Tree Search strategically explores possible moves through simulations, balancing exploration with exploitation [12, 13].

This example offers valuable insights directly applicable to the field of artificial intelligence-enhanced medical diagnostics. Like Shogi artificial intelligence, diagnostic artificial intelligence tools can objectively analyze complex medical datasets to identify patterns potentially overlooked due to human cognitive biases. Effective collaboration between health-care professionals and artificial intelligence developers is essential, ensuring these systems complement, rather than replace, human judgment. Moreover, Shogi illustrates the value of iterative learning through artificial intelligence insights, paralleling how health-care professionals can iteratively improve diagnostic accuracy by integrating artificial intelligence-generated findings into practice.

However, it is essential to recognize the contextual differences and practical considerations that distinguish this collaboration from applications in medical diagnostics. While Shogi's application of artificial intelligence is confined within a controlled game environment, artificial intelligence in medical diagnostics deals with real-life decisions with substantial consequences. Errors in diagnostics directly affect patient safety, necessitating stringent validation, ethical scrutiny, and regulatory oversight. Additionally, medical diagnostics must handle complex variables such as patient diversity and evolving medical knowledge, considerably amplifying the complexity and importance of interdisciplinary collaboration. Beyond board games, similar interdisciplinary lessons can be seen in sports such as baseball, where strategy, teamwork, and data analytics intersect in ways that parallel medical diagnostics.

12.2.2 Baseball

In the broader realm of sports, artificial intelligence has rapidly gained traction as a transformative tool, enhancing decision-making, performance analysis, and strategic planning. From basketball to tennis, artificial intelligence technologies are increasingly being used to track player movements, assess biomechanical data, and optimize training regimens. These advancements are driven by close collaboration among athletes, coaches, data scientists, and artificial intelligence engineers, emphasizing the power of interdisciplinary synergy in high-performance environments [14].

Among these sports, baseball stands out as a particularly compelling example of successful interdisciplinary collaboration between professionals and artificial intelligence developers. Artificial intelligence and data analytics have transformed baseball, improving decision-making, optimizing player performance, and redefining strategic team management. Artificial intelligence-driven analyses in baseball encompass comprehensive datasets covering player biomechanics, game statistics, and environmental variables like pitch velocity and weather conditions.

Artificial intelligence systems have empowered teams to identify subtle patterns and extract actionable insights that would otherwise remain hidden from human observers [15]. For example, the introduction of machine learning models in baseball has enabled predictive analytics for the following:

- Pitch selection: Artificial intelligence can predict an opposing pitcher's next move based on historical patterns and current game dynamics. This helps batters anticipate pitches with greater accuracy [16].
- Injury prevention: Artificial intelligence tools analyze players' movements and physiological data to detect potential injury risks early and recommend optimized training regimens [17].
- Scouting and recruitment: Artificial intelligence-driven tools assess player performance metrics and simulate future potential, enabling teams to make informed recruitment decisions [18].

One notable case is the adoption of artificial intelligence technologies in Major League Baseball [19]. These organizations have incorporated artificial intelligence-based systems to enhance player development and tactical decision-making. Technologies such as TrackMan and Statcast utilize machine learning algorithms to provide precise real-time measurements of pitch spin rates, launch angles, and player positioning. These insights enable coaching staff and players to fine-tune their techniques and strategies for optimal outcomes [20, 21].

Interdisciplinary collaboration in baseball extends beyond players and coaches to include sports scientists, data analysts, and artificial intelligence engineers. By working together, these professionals ensure that artificial intelligence systems are seamlessly integrated into team operations, leading to evidence-based decision-making and continuous improvement. For instance, wearable sensor technologies combined with machine learning algorithms offer valuable feedback on a player's physical condition, workload, and recovery needs.

In the broader context of artificial intelligence development, baseball demonstrates how the interplay between human expertise and artificial intelligence-driven analytics can produce significant performance enhancements. This successful collaboration between data science, engineering, and sports professionals serves as a model for other industries, including health care, where artificial intelligence is being adopted to optimize diagnostic accuracy and improve patient outcomes.

This example also offers valuable insights that are directly applicable to the field of artificial intelligence-enhanced medical diagnostics. The use of artificial intelligence in baseball highlights important takeaways for artificial intelligence-enhanced medical diagnostics. Just as baseball artificial intelligence tools analyze complex data to uncover hidden patterns, artificial intelligence in medical diagnostics can sift through extensive patient data to detect subtle signs of diseases and conditions that might be missed by health-care professionals. The collaboration between data scientists, coaches, and players mirrors the need for close cooperation between health-care professionals and artificial intelligence developers to ensure tools are tailored to clinical needs and practical use. Baseball also highlights the value of predictive analytics and its role in decision-making. In diagnostics, artificial intelligence's ability to predict patient risks, disease progression, or treatment outcomes can empower health-care professionals to make proactive and evidence-based decisions, improving patient care and outcomes.

However, as in the previous subsection on shogi, it is essential to recognize the contextual differences and practical considerations that distinguish this collaboration from applications in medical diagnostics. While baseball artificial intelligence focuses on performance optimization within a competitive and relatively controlled environment, artificial intelligence adoption in medical diagnostics deals with far more critical and ethically sensitive challenges. Errors in artificial intelligence-driven decisions for baseball may impact game outcomes or player performance but remain reversible; in health care, such mistakes can have direct consequences for patient health and well-being, as noted in Sect. 12.1.1.

Moreover, baseball artificial intelligence operates with highly structured and measurable data, such as player statistics, biomechanical movements, and game metrics. In contrast, artificial intelligence for diagnostics must contend with diverse, unstructured, and often incomplete datasets from medical records, imaging, and laboratory results. This complexity necessitates a higher degree of validation, transparency, and ethical oversight to ensure artificial intelligence systems in diagnostics are both accurate and trustworthy. Moving from baseball to football, the lessons become even broader, highlighting how complex, dynamic systems with multiple stakeholders can inform approaches to artificial intelligence-driven collaboration in medicine.

12.2.3 Football

In the world's most popular sport, football, commonly known as soccer, has become a fertile ground for artificial intelligence-driven transformation, fostering a deep interdisciplinary collaboration among coaches, players, medical staff, and data scientists. The sport's dynamic nature, involving 22 players in constant, fluid motion, generates vast and complex datasets, making it an ideal domain for artificial intelligence applications in tactical analysis, player performance, and injury prevention [22].

Artificial intelligence systems, powered by machine learning and computer vision, analyze data from various sources, including wearable sensors, GPS trackers, and high-definition cameras that capture every on-field action [23]. This integration of technology allows for a granular analysis of team performance and individual player metrics. For instance, artificial intelligence algorithms can:

- Optimize Tactics: By analyzing opponents' strategies and identifying weaknesses, artificial intelligence can suggest optimal formations and set-piece strategies. Google DeepMind, in collaboration with Liverpool FC, developed TacticAI, an artificial intelligence assistant that advises coaches on tactical adjustments, particularly for corner kicks [24].
- Enhance Player Performance: Artificial intelligence provides objective assessments of player skills, such as pass completion, movement patterns, and decision-making, helping coaches create personalized development plans [25].
- Prevent Injuries: One of the most significant applications of artificial intelligence in football is injury prevention. By analyzing biomechanical data, training loads, and historical injury data, artificial intelligence systems can forecast an individual player's risk of injury, allowing medical staff to intervene with preventative measures and optimized rehabilitation programs [26, 27].

This collaborative ecosystem ensures that the technological insights are both relevant and actionable. Sports scientists and medical teams work with data analysts to interpret artificial intelligence-generated risk profiles, while coaches and players use performance analytics to refine their training and in-game strategies.

The application of artificial intelligence in football offers profound lessons for medical diagnostics. The most direct parallel lies in injury prevention, where predictive artificial intelligence models in football mirror the goal of forecasting disease risk in patients based on physiological data, lifestyle factors, and medical history. Just as artificial intelligence can identify subtle patterns in a player's movement that may indicate a heightened risk of a soft-tissue injury, diagnostic artificial intelligence can detect faint signals in medical imaging or electronic health records that suggest the early onset of a condition. The collaboration among a football team's diverse staff highlights the necessity for a similar multidisciplinary approach in health care, where health-care professionals, data scientists, and ethicists must work together to translate artificial intelligence-driven insights into improved patient outcomes.

However, the stakes and complexities in medical diagnostics are fundamentally different. A flawed tactical suggestion in football might lead to a lost match, but an erroneous diagnostic prediction can have severe consequences for a patient's health and safety. The complex data in football is generated within the controlled environment of a sport with defined rules. In contrast, medical data is far more varied, often unstructured, and subject to stringent privacy regulations. Therefore, while the collaborative and data-driven strategies from football provide a valuable model, their application in medicine demands a significantly higher level of validation, ethical oversight, and consideration for the human-centric nature of patient care.

12.3 Artificial Intelligence in Medical Diagnostics: Building Interdisciplinary Collaboration

The successful integration of artificial intelligence into medical diagnostics critically depends on interdisciplinary collaboration experts from health care, computer science, data analytics, and bioethics. Unlike artificial intelligence applications in other domains, the stakes in medical diagnostics are considerably higher due to direct implications for patient safety and health outcomes. Therefore, collaboration is not only advantageous but essential for developing robust, reliable, and ethical artificial intelligence diagnostics systems.

12.3.1 Key Participants in Medical Artificial Intelligence Development

There are several key participants in artificial intelligence development in medicine as follows:

- Health-Care Professionals: Health-care professionals provide critical domain knowledge, define clinical challenges, and validate artificial intelligence outcomes. Their expertise ensures artificial intelligence systems address real-world diagnostic needs while improving workflows and patient care.
- Data Scientists and Artificial Intelligence Developers: Data scientists design and train artificial intelligence models, while developers ensure systems are efficient, scalable, and deployable in clinical settings.
- Ethicists and Legal Experts: Medical artificial intelligence raises unique ethical concerns, such as bias, data privacy, and accountability. Ethicists and legal professionals ensure compliance with regulations and ethical standards. The detailed discussion is shown in Chap. 11.
- Patients, Their Families, and Public Health Experts: Involving patient perspectives ensures artificial intelligence solutions are patient-centered, accessible, and address diverse populations' needs.
- Health-Care Administrators and Policymakers: Administrators and policymakers facilitate the adoption of artificial intelligence solutions through resource allocation, regulatory frameworks, and infrastructure development.

12.3.2 Challenges in Collaboration for Medical Artificial Intelligence

Despite the clear benefits, interdisciplinary collaboration faces several significant challenges. One major issue is the communication gap that arises when professionals from different disciplines use varied terminologies and methodologies and prioritize different goals. Overcoming this requires dedicated efforts to establish mutual understanding and shared objectives. Another challenge is data integration, as medical datasets are often fragmented, unstructured, and protected by stringent privacy laws, making it difficult to aggregate and share data for artificial intelligence model development. Furthermore, trust and adoption remain barriers, with health-care professionals sometimes hesitant to embrace artificial intelligence technologies due to concerns about transparency, accuracy, or perceived threats to their professional autonomy. Ethical and legal complexities also persist, as developers must ensure that artificial intelligence systems remain transparent, accountable, ethically sound, and compliant with all relevant regulations.

12.3.3 Strategies for Effective Collaboration

To address these collaborative challenges, several strategies can be implemented. Cross-disciplinary education is essential, requiring health-care professionals to gain foundational knowledge in artificial intelligence and the developers to acquire clinical context, thereby bridging crucial knowledge gaps—a key objective of this book. Establishing consistent interdisciplinary communication through structured meetings and collaborative workshops helps ensure ongoing dialogue and input at all stages of artificial intelligence system development and deployment. Implementing pilot programs within specific medical areas provides an opportunity to evaluate the feasibility, effectiveness, and integration of artificial intelligence solutions before full-scale implementation. Moreover, involving dedicated ethics committees throughout the artificial intelligence development lifecycle ensures continuous ethical review, promoting transparency, privacy, fairness, and accountability.

12.3.4 Learning from Other Industries

Industries such as shogi, baseball, and football offer valuable insights into effective artificial intelligence collaboration strategies that can be applied to medical diagnostics. The development of artificial intelligence in shogi revealed how an unbiased partner—free from the cognitive biases discussed in Chap. 1—can provide novel strategic insights that go beyond human cognitive biases, a benefit that similarly applies to identifying hidden diagnostic patterns in health care. The use of predictive analytics in baseball demonstrates how medical artificial intelligence can forecast disease progression and support optimized clinical decision-making, ultimately enabling more personalized care. All industries also emphasize the importance of iterative development and continuous learning, with human professionals using artificial intelligence-driven feedback to refine their expertise—an approach equally vital in health-care settings.

Nonetheless, the ethical considerations, complexity of data, and variability of clinical environments make artificial intelligence in medical diagnostics distinctively challenging. Therefore, success in this field requires rigorous validation, the cultivation of interdisciplinary trust, and the establishment of clear, ethical frameworks to ensure that artificial intelligence-driven diagnostic tools are safe, effective, and equitable.

References

1. Joksimovic S, Ifenthaler D, Marrone R, De Laat M, Siemens G. Opportunities of artificial intelligence for supporting complex problem-solving: findings from a scoping review. Comput Educ Artif Intell. 2023;4:100138.
2. Richardson JP, Smith C, Curtis S, Watson S, Zhu X, Barry B, et al. Patient apprehensions about the use of artificial intelligence in healthcare. NPJ Digit Med. 2021;4(1):140.
3. Virvou M. Artificial intelligence and user experience in reciprocity: contributions and state of the art. Intell Decision Technol. 2023;17:73–125.
4. Vesnic-Alujevic L, Nascimento S, Polvora A. Societal and ethical impacts of artificial intelligence: critical notes on European policy frameworks. Telecommun Policy. 2020;44(6):101961.
5. Corfmat M, Martineau JT, Régis C. High-reward, high-risk technologies? An ethical and legal account of AI development in healthcare. BMC Med Ethics. 2025;26(1):4.
6. Iida H, Sakuta M, Rollason J. Computer shogi. Artif Intell. 2002;134(1):121–44.
7. Matake K. Shogi and artificial intelligence. Japan policy forum Culture; 2016.
8. Matsubara H, Iida H, Grimbergen R. Natural developments in game research: from chess to shogi to go. London, England: SAGE Publications Sage UK; 1996.
9. Editorial Board TSS. Sota Fujii leads the transformation of shogi with all 8 major titles. The Sankei Shimbun 2023 October 16.
10. Shiohara T, Mizukawa Y. Ask not what AI can do to us, but what we can do with AI. J Allergy Clin Immunol Pract. 2022;10(1):284–5.
11. Schrittwieser J, Antonoglou I, Hubert T, Simonyan K, Sifre L, Schmitt S, et al. Mastering atari, go, chess and shogi by planning with a learned model. Nature. 2020;588(7839):604–9.
12. Gonzalez K. Enhanced Monte Carlo tree search in game-playing AI: evaluating Deepmind's algorithms. 2023.
13. Silver D, Hubert T, Schrittwieser J, Antonoglou I, Lai M, Guez A, et al. A general reinforcement learning algorithm that masters chess, shogi, and go through self-play. Science (New York, NY). 2018;362(6419):1140–4.
14. Ghosh I, Ramasamy Ramamurthy S, Chakma A, Roy N. Sports analytics review: artificial intelligence applications, emerging technologies, and algorithmic perspective. WIREs Data Min Knowl Discov. 2023;13(5):e1496.
15. Davis J, Bransen L, Devos L, Jaspers A, Meert W, Robberechts P, et al. Methodology and evaluation in sports analytics: challenges, approaches, and lessons learned. Mach Learn. 2024;113(9):6977–7010.
16. Ashok M, Madan R, Joha A, Sivarajah U. Ethical framework for artificial intelligence and digital technologies. Int J Inf Manag. 2022;62:102433.
17. Claudino JG, Capanema DO, de Souza TV, Serrão JC, Machado Pereira AC, Nassis GP. Current approaches to the use of artificial intelligence for injury risk assessment and performance prediction in team sports: a systematic review. Sports Med Open. 2019;5(1):28.
18. Xu T, Baghaei S. Reshaping the future of sports with artificial intelligence: challenges and opportunities in performance enhancement, fan engagement, and strategic decision-making. Eng Appl Artif Intell. 2025;142:109912.
19. Koseler K, Stephan M. Machine learning applications in baseball: a systematic literature review. Appl Artif Intell. 2017;31(9–10):745–63.
20. Healey G. The new Moneyball: how ballpark sensors are changing baseball. Proc IEEE. 2017;105(11):1999–2002.
21. Nathan AM, editor Analysis of Baseball Trajectories. Physics; 2017.

22. Beal R, Norman TJ, Ramchurn SD. Artificial intelligence for team sports: a survey. Knowl Eng Rev. 2019;34:e28.
23. Yang T, Yuan G, Yan J. Health analysis of footballer using big data and deep learning. Sci Program. 2021;2021(1):9608147.
24. Wang Z, Veličković P, Hennes D, Tomašev N, Prince L, Kaisers M, et al. TacticAI: an AI assistant for football tactics. Nat Commun. 2024;15(1):1906.
25. Liao S, Fu C. The optimization of youth football training using deep learning and artificial intelligence. Sci Rep. 2025;15(1):8190.
26. Van Eetvelde H, Mendonça LD, Ley C, Seil R, Tischer T. Machine learning methods in sport injury prediction and prevention: a systematic review. J Exp Orthop. 2021;8(1):27.
27. Nassis GP, Verhagen E, Brito J, Figueiredo P, Krustrup P. A review of machine learning applications in soccer with an emphasis on injury risk. Biol Sport. 2023;40(1):233–9.

Challenges and Solutions in AI Deployment

13

Abstract

This chapter addresses the practical challenges encountered when deploying artificial intelligence systems and outlines viable solutions. The chapter discusses technical, organizational, ethical, and regulatory issues, providing comprehensive strategies for overcoming these hurdles. This chapter also includes an expanded exploration of historical contexts, detailed case studies, and methodological guidance aligned with the human-organization-technology fit framework to ensure holistic and effective integration.

Keywords

Artificial intelligence deployment · Healthcare challenges · Data quality · Algorithm bias · Workflow integration · Ethical concerns · Regulatory frameworks · Human · Organization · Technology fit framework

13.1 Overview of Challenges and Solutions

Deploying artificial intelligence in health care has the potential to significantly enhance diagnostics, treatment personalization, and operational efficiency. However, numerous challenges exist at the intersection of technology, infrastructure, regulation, and human factors. This chapter examines these challenges and provides practical solutions guided by the human-organization-technology (HOT) fit framework [1], illustrated in Fig. 13.1. The following sections provide a detailed exploration of each dimension with specific real-world examples, strategies, and outcomes.

T. Hirosawa, *Artificial Intelligence in Medical Diagnostics*,
https://doi.org/10.1007/978-981-95-4338-0_13

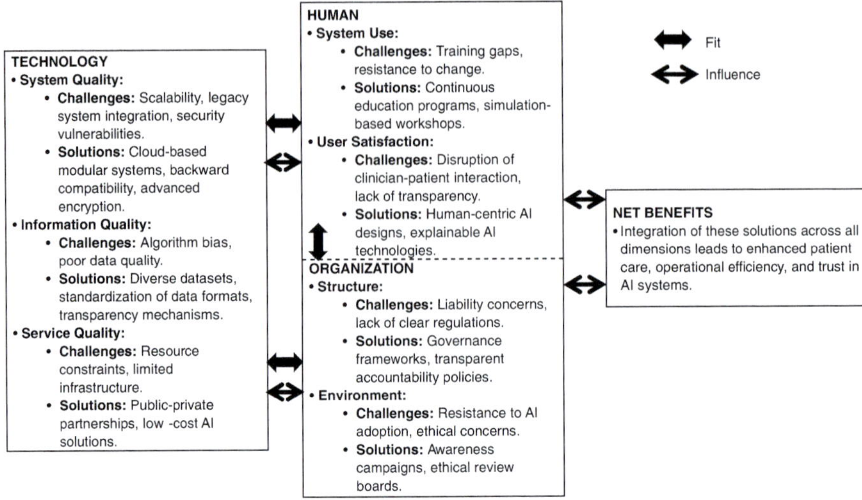

Fig. 13.1 Proposed human-organization-technology (HOT fit) fit framework adapted to reflect the current context of integrating artificial intelligence (AI) systems

13.2 Clinical and User-Focused Challenges and Solutions

This section addresses critical challenges in artificial intelligence deployment within health care, including inadequate professional training, disruptions in health-care professional-patient interactions, workflow inefficiencies, and uncertainties surrounding liability. It also proposes targeted solutions emphasizing education, human-centric artificial intelligence design, systematic workflow integration, and clear governance frameworks to ensure effective and sustainable artificial intelligence adoption.

13.2.1 Training and Education for Health-Care Professionals

A critical challenge is the lack of sufficient training and education among health-care professionals in artificial intelligence applications, often leading to its under-utilization or misapplication [2]. Historically, limited educational offerings have created significant knowledge gaps, resulting in suboptimal implementation and apprehension among health-care professionals.

To address this, continuous education programs specifically tailored to health-care professionals are essential [3, 4]. These programs should combine theoretical knowledge with practical skills, covering artificial intelligence fundamentals, clinical applications, ethical considerations, and hands-on simulation-based workshops [2]. Collaborations among educational institutions, industry partners, and certification bodies can facilitate comprehensive and targeted training, accelerating adoption and ensuring sustained utilization.

Such initiatives have been shown to significantly enhance health-care professionals' confidence, promote effective artificial intelligence utilization, and improve patient outcomes. Further details on education and training strategies are provided in Chap. 14.

13.2.2 Health-Care Professional-Patient Interaction

Artificial intelligence deployment can potentially disrupt the interaction between health-care professionals and patients, risking reduced patient satisfaction and trust. For example, erroneous artificial intelligence-driven diagnoses accessed directly by patients could lead to serious health consequences, highlighting the need for cautious integration [5].

The solution lies in designing artificial intelligence systems that complement rather than replace health-care professionals [6]. Artificial intelligence developers should emphasize human-centric designs, empowering health-care professionals to leverage artificial intelligence without compromising their professional decision-making [7]. Health-care professionals should also receive specialized training to effectively incorporate artificial intelligence into their practice, ensuring clear and empathetic patient communication, thereby maintaining trust and enhancing interaction quality. Strategies such as interactive patient education tools and collaborative decision-making frameworks further reinforce trust, patient satisfaction, and acceptance of artificial intelligence-enhanced care.

13.2.3 Workflow Disruption

Integrating artificial intelligence into established clinical workflows often results in temporary inefficiencies and professional resistance. Increased workloads from adopting new technologies have historically hindered health-care professionals' acceptance and satisfaction [8]. For example, a new artificial intelligence diagnostic tool requires health-care professionals to enter data into a separate interface outside of the main electronic health record, disrupting clinical flow and leading to frustration. Such disruption can negatively impact overall productivity if not adequately addressed.

To mitigate this, systematic workflow assessments must be conducted to identify potential disruptions before full deployment. Engaging health-care professionals early and directly in artificial intelligence design and development fosters tailored solutions compatible with existing practices. Additionally, implementing pilot programs and adopting iterative feedback loops ensure incremental, smooth integration, minimizing disruptions, and enhancing workflow efficiency. Examples from various clinical environments illustrate the effectiveness of phased implementation, continuous monitoring, and adaptation based on health-care professionals' feedback.

13.2.4 Liability and Accountability

The complexity introduced by artificial intelligence in clinical decision-making generates uncertainty around liability and accountability, often causing hesitation among health-care professionals to adopt artificial intelligence [9]. This uncertainty can also complicate regulatory compliance and malpractice risk management.

To overcome this challenge, clear policies and collaborative governance frameworks must be established to explicitly delineate the responsibilities of health-care professionals and artificial intelligence developers [10]. Implementing transparent and well-documented processes, conducting regular performance audits, and promoting international harmonization of accountability standards can clarify roles and responsibilities [11]. This approach reduces liability concerns, enhances transparency, and increases health-care professionals' confidence in artificial intelligence systems. Case studies from jurisdictions successfully integrating comprehensive governance frameworks provide practical insights into managing liability and accountability effectively.

13.3 Technical Challenges and Solutions

13.3.1 Data Quality and Accessibility

Artificial intelligence effectiveness in health care critically depends on the availability and quality of data. Common barriers include inadequate data quality, inconsistent formatting, and limited data-sharing capabilities across institutions. Historically, health-care data has often been collected through methods prone to errors, such as handwritten notes, fragmented legacy systems, and electronic health records operating on incompatible platforms, significantly hindering interoperability and comprehensive data usage [12].

To overcome these challenges, health-care institutions should actively prioritize data standardization initiatives. This includes implementing robust interoperability frameworks and adopting universally recognized data standards, such as Health Level Seven International® Fast Healthcare Interoperability Resources® (HL7 FHIR®) [13]. Real-time data collection systems, automated data verification tools, and streamlined, secured data-sharing protocols across diverse health-care institutions are essential to ensure artificial intelligence models receive accurate and reliable input data, ultimately enhancing predictive accuracy and clinical reliability [14]. International initiatives demonstrating successful interoperability, such as the European eHealth Digital Service Infrastructure, offer valuable reference models that institutions globally can replicate to facilitate seamless data integration and sharing [15, 16].

13.3.2 Algorithm Bias and Fairness

Algorithmic bias in artificial intelligence systems presents a critical challenge, often resulting in health-care disparities, particularly among underrepresented and minority populations [17]. Bias typically arises from skewed training datasets disproportionately representing affluent, predominantly English-speaking populations, thereby inadequately reflecting conditions prevalent in economically disadvantaged or culturally diverse communities.

A pertinent example includes neglected tropical diseases, prevalent in low-resource regions. Due to insufficient representation in mainstream datasets, predictive algorithms frequently underperform or provide inaccurate diagnoses for these populations, exacerbating existing health-care disparities [18]. Additionally, cultural factors such as variations in health-care-seeking behaviors and symptom reporting further skew algorithmic outputs, potentially leading to misdiagnoses or inappropriate treatment recommendations.

To mitigate these biases, institutions must implement regular and rigorous algorithmic auditing processes alongside advanced bias detection methods. Deliberately incorporating diverse and representative datasets during the artificial intelligence training phase is critical for enhancing algorithmic fairness and accuracy. Transparency through publicly available reporting on datasets and artificial intelligence model performance, alongside iterative algorithm updates informed by continuous real-world monitoring, promotes ethical artificial intelligence development and equitable health-care outcomes.

13.3.3 Scalability and Infrastructure

Scalability remains a significant hurdle in the widespread implementation of artificial intelligence in health care, primarily due to limited computational infrastructure and resources within many health-care institutions. Historically, the costs and complexities associated with establishing robust artificial intelligence infrastructure have created substantial barriers to adoption, particularly for small and medium-sized enterprises [19].

Health-care organizations should explore adopting scalable, cloud-based solutions and modular artificial intelligence frameworks, enabling incremental infrastructure enhancements tailored to specific institutional requirements and growth trajectories. Cloud solutions provide flexibility, cost-effectiveness, and scalability advantages, facilitating more efficient resource allocation and reducing the burden on local information technology infrastructures [20]. Detailed cost-benefit analyses comparing cloud versus on-premises solutions can effectively guide health-care institutions in making informed, strategic investment decisions for sustainable and scalable artificial intelligence deployments. Alongside infrastructure concerns, safeguarding security and privacy is equally critical in health-care artificial intelligence deployment.

13.3.4 Security and Privacy

Artificial intelligence deployment in health care introduces heightened security and privacy risks due to the sensitivity of patient health data [21]. Historical security breaches highlight the urgent necessity for advanced, proactive security measures to safeguard data integrity and patient confidentiality [22].

To address these risks, health-care organizations must rigorously implement encryption technologies and secure data management protocols and privacy-preserving methodologies such as federated learning and differential privacy [23]. Regular and comprehensive security audits, combined with robust continuous monitoring systems, are essential for promptly identifying, assessing, and addressing vulnerabilities and potential threats. Establishing stringent data governance frameworks, reinforced by stringent regulatory compliance and patient-centric privacy policies, further fortifies data security and trust in artificial intelligence systems. These essential security and privacy concerns are discussed in greater detail in Chap. 11.

13.4 Organizational Challenges and Solutions

Effective integration of artificial intelligence into health-care systems requires addressing several organizational challenges. Resistance to change, integration complexities with existing systems, and resource constraints are prominent issues that must be strategically managed to ensure successful and sustainable adoption.

13.4.1 Resistance to Change

Resistance from health-care professionals and administrators to adopting artificial intelligence technologies often arises from skepticism, fear of losing autonomy in clinical decision-making, and concerns about workflow disruptions [8, 24]. Historically, such resistance has led to delayed implementation and limited effectiveness in achieving anticipated outcomes from technological innovations.

To address these concerns, comprehensive change management strategies should be implemented, including structured training programs to increase familiarity and comfort with artificial intelligence technologies. Clear and consistent communication emphasizing the clinical and operational benefits of artificial intelligence can mitigate misconceptions and build trust. Direct involvement of health-care professionals and administrators in pilot projects allows stakeholders to actively experience the potential improvements artificial intelligence can offer, fostering acceptance through demonstrated results. Setting explicit adoption milestones, monitoring measurable success indicators, and providing ongoing support throughout transition phases are critical in achieving sustained and successful artificial intelligence integration.

13.4.2 Integration with Existing Systems

Integrating artificial intelligence technologies into existing legacy health information systems often encounters compatibility issues, presenting significant challenges that historically impede efficient adoption [25]. Common issues include data interoperability constraints, outdated software infrastructure, and lack of system flexibility.

To overcome these integration barriers, it is essential to design artificial intelligence solutions with backward compatibility in mind. Employing middleware, application programming interfaces, and custom integration software can significantly enhance compatibility, enabling seamless interaction between new artificial intelligence applications and legacy systems. Moreover, actively involving end-users, particularly health-care professionals and administrative personnel, during the development and integration phases ensures that solutions meet practical needs, reducing friction during adoption and facilitating smoother operational transitions.

13.4.3 Resource Constraints

Adopting artificial intelligence technologies in resource-constrained health-care settings presents significant challenges, including financial limitations, inadequate technological infrastructure, and limited human resources skilled in artificial intelligence deployment and management. These constraints have historically restricted the accessibility of advanced technological solutions, thereby widening the divide in health care [26].

To effectively address these constraints, establishing public-private partnerships can mobilize financial and technical resources, making artificial intelligence adoption economically feasible for resource-limited environments. Utilizing low-cost or open-source artificial intelligence solutions reduces financial barriers and provides scalable options for implementation [27]. Additionally, fostering international collaborations allows for the exchange of expertise, resources, and technology tailored specifically to the needs of resource-constrained settings. Case studies highlighting successful artificial intelligence implementations in similar contexts serve as practical blueprints, offering valuable insights and proven strategies for replication and adaptation [28]. Training local personnel in artificial intelligence management through capacity-building initiatives further ensures sustainable technology utilization and long term operational effectiveness.

13.5 Ethical and Regulatory Challenges and Solutions

As an organizational factor in the HOT fit framework, ethical and regulatory concerns play a critical role in influencing the adoption and integration of artificial intelligence in health care, including medical diagnostics. The absence of standardized guidelines poses significant challenges, leading to inconsistencies and uncertainties in artificial intelligence implementation across health-care sectors. Moreover, limited transparency in artificial intelligence decision-making processes generates ethical apprehensions among stakeholders, including patients, health-care professionals, and regulators [29, 30].

To mitigate these challenges, health-care institutions and policymakers must collaboratively develop robust regulatory frameworks that emphasize patient safety, equitable access, fairness, and transparency. Establishing clear standards and guidelines provides essential benchmarks for artificial intelligence technology developers and users, ensuring compliance with ethical norms and legal requirements. Forming dedicated ethical review boards with explicit operational guidelines and oversight functions can critically evaluate artificial intelligence solutions and their implications for patient care, ensuring adherence to ethical practices and responsible innovation [31].

Current regulatory shifts—such as moves to classify certain digital health-care applications as medical devices—open the possibility for systematic reporting and oversight of artificial intelligence-related incidents [32]. This development establishes a foundation for more robust accountability mechanisms and aligns artificial intelligence use in health care with established patient safety protocols traditionally applied to medical technologies.

Promoting transparency through explainable artificial intelligence technologies is essential to build trust among health-care professionals, patients, and other stakeholders. Explainability in artificial intelligence ensures that decision-making processes can be clearly understood and justified, reducing fears surrounding accountability and liability [33]. Stakeholder education programs, targeted communication campaigns, and training on ethical artificial intelligence usage further enhance acceptance and integration.

Additionally, regular audits and continuous monitoring of artificial intelligence systems should be mandated to ensure sustained adherence to ethical standards and regulatory compliance [11]. Encouraging active engagement and feedback from various stakeholders, including patients, health-care professionals, policymakers, and technology developers, fosters an inclusive approach to artificial intelligence governance, promoting solutions that are both ethical and practically beneficial [10]. Detailed ethical and regulatory considerations in artificial intelligence diagnostics are further elaborated in Chap. 11.

13.6 Case Studies and Best Practices

Real-world examples where artificial intelligence deployment encountered significant challenges can provide valuable insights. Case studies such as the deployment of artificial intelligence in resource-constrained hospitals, addressing bias in diagnostic algorithms, and successfully scaling artificial intelligence systems across multiple health-care facilities are essential to understanding effective solutions. Detailed case studies in artificial intelligence-enhanced diagnostics are discussed in Chap. 9.

13.7 Future Outlook

The future landscape of artificial intelligence deployment in medical diagnostics is characterized by increasing integration and complex challenges, which will redefine roles for policymakers, developers, and health-care professionals. Emerging trends include advancements in precision medicine driven by sophisticated artificial intelligence algorithms, growing reliance on personalized diagnostic insights, and proactive rather than reactive health-care strategies.

Continuous innovation is crucial, necessitating ongoing investment in artificial intelligence research and development. Anticipating and proactively addressing emerging ethical, technical, and regulatory challenges will facilitate smooth integration. Forward-looking strategies should emphasize collaborative governance models involving multiple stakeholders, thus ensuring artificial intelligence solutions are both ethically robust and practically advantageous technologies. Chapter 15 further elaborates on anticipated developments, potential barriers, and strategic recommendations for sustained, effective, and equitable integration of artificial intelligence technologies into health-care practices.

In summary, systematic and collaborative approaches that encompass technical, ethical, organizational and regulatory dimensions are essential to address the inherent challenges in artificial intelligence-driven diagnostics. This integrated strategy ensures artificial intelligence's potential is fully realized, contributing to enhanced health-care delivery and equitable outcomes.

References

1. Yusof MM, Kuljis J, Papazafeiropoulou A, Stergioulas LK. An evaluation framework for Health Information Systems: human, organization and technology-fit factors (HOT-fit). Int J Med Inform. 2008;77(6):386–98.
2. Southworth J, Migliaccio K, Glover J, Glover JN, Reed D, McCarty C, et al. Developing a model for AI Across the curriculum: transforming the higher education landscape via innovation in AI literacy. Comput Educ Artif Intell. 2023;4:100127.
3. Baturalp TB, Bozkurt S, Baldock C. The future of biomedical engineering education is transdisciplinary. Phys Eng Sci Med. 2024:1–4.
4. Laupichler MC, Aster A, Schirch J, Raupach T. Artificial intelligence literacy in higher and adult education: a scoping literature review. Comput Educ Artif Intell. 2022;3:100101.
5. Saenger JA, Hunger J, Boss A, Richter J. Delayed diagnosis of a transient ischemic attack caused by ChatGPT. Wien Klin Wochenschr. 2024;136(7-8):236–8.
6. Karches KE. Against the iDoctor: why artificial intelligence should not replace physician judgment. Theor Med Bioethics. 2018;39(2):91–110.
7. Rožanec JM, Inna N, Patrik Z, Klemen K, Hooman TG, Sungho S, et al. Human-centric artificial intelligence architecture for industry 5.0 applications. Int J Prod Res. 2023;61(20):6847–72.
8. Meunier PY, Raynaud C, Guimaraes E, Gueyffier F, Letrilliart L. Barriers and facilitators to the use of clinical decision support systems in primary care: a mixed-methods systematic review. Ann Fam Med. 2023;21(1):57–69.
9. Jones C, Thornton J, Wyatt JC. Artificial intelligence and clinical decision support: clinicians' perspectives on trust, trustworthiness, and liability. Med Law Rev. 2023;31(4):501–20.
10. Taeihagh A. Governance of artificial intelligence. Polic Soc. 2021;40(2):137–57.

11. Cihon P, Maas MM, Kemp L. Fragmentation and the future: investigating architectures for international AI governance. Glob Policy. 2020;11(5):545–56.
12. Alpert JS. The electronic medical record in 2016: advantages and disadvantages. Digit Med. 2016;2(2)
13. Duda SN, Kennedy N, Conway D, Cheng AC, Nguyen V, Zayas-Cabán T, et al. HL7 FHIR-based tools and initiatives to support clinical research: a scoping review. J Am Med Inform Assoc. 2022;29(9):1642–53.
14. Saleem JJ, Herout J, editors. Transitioning from one electronic health record (EHR) to another: a narrative literature review. Proceedings of the Human Factors and Ergonomics Society annual meeting. Los Angeles: Sage; 2018.
15. Dash S, Shakyawar SK, Sharma M, Kaushik S. Big data in healthcare: management, analysis and future prospects. J Big Data. 2019;6(1):54.
16. Bruthans J, Jiráková K. the current state and usage of European electronic cross-border health services (eHDSI). J Med Syst. 2023;47(1):21.
17. Panch T, Mattie H, Atun R. Artificial intelligence and algorithmic bias: implications for health systems. J Glob Health. 2019;9(2):010318.
18. Feasey N, Wansbrough-Jones M, Mabey DCW, Solomon AW. Neglected tropical diseases. Br Med Bull. 2009;93(1):179–200.
19. Rajaram K, Tinguely PN. Generative artificial intelligence in small and medium enterprises: navigating its promises and challenges. Bus Horizons. 2024;67(5):629–48.
20. Manvi SS, Krishna SG. Resource management for Infrastructure as a Service (IaaS) in cloud computing: a survey. J Netw Comput Appl. 2014;41:424–40.
21. Price WN 2nd, Cohen IG. Privacy in the age of medical big data. Nat Med. 2019;25(1):37–43.
22. Markos E, Peña P, Labrecque LI, Swani K. Are data breaches the new norm? Exploring data breach trends, consumer sentiment, and responses to security invasions. J Consum Aff. 2023;57(3):1089–119.
23. Murdoch B. Privacy and artificial intelligence: challenges for protecting health information in a new era. BMC Med Ethics. 2021;22(1):122.
24. Vanagas G, Engelbrecht R, Damaševičius R, Suomi R, Solanas A. eHealth solutions for the Integrated Healthcare. J Healthc Eng. 2018;2018:3846892.
25. Forcier MB, Gallois H, Mullan S, Joly Y. Integrating artificial intelligence into health care through data access: can the GDPR act as a beacon for policymakers? J Law Biosci. 2019;6(1):317–35.
26. Kiyasseh D, Zhu T, Clifton D. The promise of clinical decision support systems targetting low-resource settings. IEEE Rev Biomed Eng. 2022;15:354–71.
27. Erion G, Janizek JD, Hudelson C, Utarnachitt RB, McCoy AM, Sayre MR, et al. A cost-aware framework for the development of AI models for healthcare applications. Nat Biomed Eng. 2022;6(12):1384–98.
28. Schwalbe N, Wahl B. Artificial intelligence and the future of global health. Lancet. 2020;395(10236):1579–86.
29. Mennella C, Maniscalco U, De Pietro G, Esposito M. Ethical and regulatory challenges of AI technologies in healthcare: a narrative review. Heliyon. 2024;10(4):e26297.
30. Wirtz BW, Weyerer JC, Sturm BJ. The dark sides of artificial intelligence: an integrated AI governance framework for public administration. Int J Public Adm. 2020;43(9):818–29.
31. WHO. Ethics and governance of artificial intelligence for health. WHO Guidance; 2021.
32. Pruski M. AI-Enhanced Healthcare: Not a new Paradigm for Informed Consent. J Bioethical Inquiry. 2024;21(3):475–89.
33. Angelov PP, Soares EA, Jiang R, Arnold NI, Atkinson PM. Explainable artificial intelligence: an analytical review. Wiley Interdiscip Rev Data Mining Knowl Discov. 2021;11(5):e1424.

Training and Education for AI in Health Care

14

Abstract

The integration of artificial intelligence in health care is advancing rapidly, promising improvements in medical diagnostics, patient care, and administrative efficiency. To realize these benefits, health-care professionals must receive comprehensive training and education in digital health, including artificial intelligence. This chapter examines the importance of artificial intelligence literacy, outlines the necessity of targeted education for health-care professionals, and discusses curriculum development strategies aimed at bridging current knowledge gaps.

Keywords

Artificial intelligence literacy · Digital literacy · Medical education · Curriculum development · Diagnostic training

14.1 Educational Paradigm Shift

Educational methodologies historically reflect societal and technological transformations—from oral storytelling traditions to technology-enhanced learning [1]. The conventional knowledge-based educational style, which emphasizes standardized testing, is becoming increasingly obsolete in a world where artificial intelligence automates routine tasks [2]. Future-oriented education must foster critical thinking, creativity, adaptability, and a thorough understanding of digital health, including the capabilities of artificial intelligence, limitations, and ethical implications in medical contexts.

T. Hirosawa, *Artificial Intelligence in Medical Diagnostics*,
https://doi.org/10.1007/978-981-95-4338-0_14

14.1.1 Digital Literacy

Digital literacy, introduced by Paul Gilster, forms the foundational skill set required to navigate contemporary technological landscapes [3]. It encompasses competencies necessary for effectively utilizing digital tools, critically evaluating online information, and adapting to emerging technologies [4]. In the health-care sector, digital literacy ensures that health-care professionals can competently and confidently engage with technologies underpinning artificial intelligence applications, thereby enhancing their operational effectiveness in clinical environments [5].

14.1.2 Artificial Intelligence Literacy

Artificial intelligence literacy builds upon digital literacy by providing specialized competencies critical to evaluating, utilizing, and collaborating with artificial intelligence technologies. Artificial intelligence literacy is defined as "a set of competencies that enables individuals to critically evaluate artificial intelligence technologies, communicate and collaborate effectively with artificial intelligence, and use artificial intelligence as a tool online, at home, and in the workplace" [6]. Bridging the gap between artificial intelligence developers and health-care professionals requires cultivating artificial intelligence literacy for health-care professionals to facilitate mutual understanding, effective collaboration, and optimized use of artificial intelligence systems, as discussed extensively in Chap. 6.

14.1.3 Five Core Literacies in Artificial Intelligence

While digital literacy has expanded to encompass multiple new literacies, including artificial intelligence literacy [7], Davy Tsz Kit Ng et al. propose that artificial intelligence literacy comprises five core literacies [8]. First, enabling artificial intelligence refers to a foundational understanding of artificial intelligence fundamentals, including machine learning, data management, and algorithm design. Second, knowing and understanding artificial intelligence involves grasping both its theoretical foundations and practical implications. This includes recognizing technology's potential applications across medical diagnostics. It also requires an awareness of its current capabilities in clinical support and necessitates understanding inherent limitations such as data dependency, algorithmic bias, and contextual sensitivity. Third, using and applying artificial intelligence focuses on deploying artificial intelligence tools effectively in practical scenarios, enhancing real-world problem-solving capabilities. Fourth, evaluating and creating artificial intelligence includes critically assessing artificial intelligence outputs and innovatively developing new solutions. Finally, ethical considerations address the implications of artificial intelligence, highlighting responsibilities regarding ethical usage, bias recognition, and transparency. These literacies are vital for developing a proficient workforce capable of integrating artificial intelligence seamlessly into clinical practices. In 2022,

Laupichler et al. reviewed 30 studies describing how artificial intelligence literacy was being taught in higher education. They found the research to be in its infancy and identified the need for refinement of concepts and materials. In addition, none of these reviewed studies portrayed campus-wide initiatives [9].

As health-care professionals increasingly use and apply artificial intelligence, developing practical skills for deploying artificial intelligence tools in real-world scenarios becomes essential. Specifically, practical skills include techniques such as reverse prompt engineering, which involves analyzing an artificial intelligence's outputs to deduce the most effective way to phrase an input or prompt [10]. By working backward from the artificial intelligence's response, health-care professionals can learn to refine their queries, enhancing the accuracy and reliability of the generated recommendations and reducing errors [11].

14.1.4 Adapting Core Literacy in Generative Artificial Intelligence

In generative artificial intelligence contexts, these core literacies are tailored to emphasize knowledge of generative models, including neural network structures and training mechanisms such as transformer architectures. Health-care professionals must understand generative artificial intelligence's diverse applications, gain practical experience in fine-tuning and deploying generative models, critically evaluate outputs, and address ethical considerations, including the responsible management of misinformation and intellectual property. These adapted competencies ensure effective use and integration of generative artificial intelligence technologies in health care, detailed in Table 14.1.

Table 14.1 Comparing general artificial intelligence literacy and generative artificial intelligence literacy

Literacy	Artificial intelligence literacy	Generative artificial intelligence literacy
1. Enabling	Foundational knowledge of artificial intelligence principles: machine learning, data processing, algorithm design	Foundational knowledge of generative models: neural architectures, training mechanisms (e.g., transformers)
2. Knowing & understanding	Awareness of artificial intelligence capabilities, limitations, and applications	Awareness of generative artificial intelligence capabilities, limitations, and applications (text, image, content creation)
3. Using & applying	Practical skills in deploying artificial intelligence tools in real-world scenarios	Hands on experience of platforms; fine-tuning and deploying pre-trained generative models
4. Evaluating	Assessment of artificial intelligence outputs for quality, biases, and solution development	Assessment of generative outputs for relevance, quality, biases, and performance
5. Ethical considerations	Ethical awareness of bias, responsibility, and implications in health care	Responsible use of generative artificial intelligence: transparency, risk mitigation (misinformation, intellectual property infringement)

14.2 Necessity of Artificial Intelligence Education in Medical Diagnostics

As artificial intelligence-driven medical diagnostic tools become common in the near future, health-care professionals must be able to evaluate the validity, reliability, and practicality. Education in artificial intelligence equips health-care professionals with the skills necessary to collaborate effectively with developers, recognize artificial intelligence limitations, and use artificial intelligence insights to minimize diagnostic errors and optimize patient outcomes. Addressing knowledge gaps through targeted education mitigates risks associated with artificial intelligence misuse and underutilization, as discussed further in Chap. 7.

Effective integration of artificial intelligence in medical diagnostics requires seamless collaboration between artificial intelligence developers and health-care professionals. Often, there exists a significant gap in mutual understanding between these two groups due to differences in background, expertise, terminology, and objectives. Artificial intelligence developers mainly focus on technical performance and algorithmic efficiency, while health-care professionals prioritize clinical relevance, patient safety, and usability in real-world scenarios. Bridging this gap necessitates interdisciplinary communication strategies, such as collaborative workshops, seminars, and regular dialogue forums, which foster mutual understanding and encourage co-creation of artificial intelligence solutions tailored specifically to clinical environments. Encouraging artificial intelligence developers to participate in clinical rotations or observational sessions can significantly enhance their appreciation of the health-care context, leading to more practical, efficient, and patient-oriented artificial intelligence tools. Interdisciplinary collaboration for artificial intelligence development is detailed in Chap. 12.

14.3 Curriculum Development for Artificial Intelligence in Health Care

A structured artificial intelligence curriculum tailored specifically to health-care professionals is crucial. Current artificial intelligence education resources are often fragmented and lack a health-care perspective [12].

14.3.1 Key Components of Artificial Intelligence Curriculum in Health Care

Key components include introductory modules that cover the basics of artificial intelligence, including historical context, core principles, and current applications in health care. Technical training should provide hands-on experience with artificial intelligence tools, such as machine learning platforms, natural language processing, and computer vision technologies. Case studies featuring real-world examples of artificial intelligence successes and failures in medical diagnostics offer insights into best practices [13]. Ethics and legal considerations should be an integral part of the curriculum, with training on regulatory compliance, patient data privacy, and ethical dilemmas [14, 15]. Interdisciplinary collaboration can be fostered through workshops and seminars that bring together health-care professionals, technologists, and artificial intelligence developers [16]. Standardized assessments and certifications can measure artificial intelligence proficiency and readiness for clinical integration. These components are designed to directly build the five core literacies: introductory modules address "Enabling" artificial intelligence; case studies and technical training address "Knowing, Understanding, Using, and Applying"; ethics and legal training address "Ethical Considerations"; and a focus on interdisciplinary collaboration supports the innovative "Evaluating and Creating" literacy.

14.3.2 Implementing the Artificial Intelligence Curriculum: Challenges and Solutions

Implementing a robust artificial intelligence-focused curriculum within the health-care domain presents multiple challenges [17]. First, there are substantial limitations, including insufficient funding, inadequate infrastructure, and lack of access to high-quality digital tools essential for teaching artificial intelligence [18]. Second, a critical shortage of qualified instructors who possess expertise in both artificial intelligence technologies and health-care practices creates a barrier to delivering contextually relevant instruction [19]. Third, learners exhibit varied levels of prior exposure to digital technologies and artificial intelligence concepts [20], necessitating differentiated instructional approaches.

To address these issues, institutions can adopt hybrid learning models that combine online content with in-person workshops or practical training sessions. This blended approach provides flexibility and fosters hands-on experience with artificial intelligence tools. Partnerships with universities, hospitals, and technology companies can supply expert resources, enhance content relevance, and promote cross-sector collaboration. Establishing standardized training programs for instructors ensures consistent delivery of artificial intelligence education and facilitates capacity building. Additionally, integrating adaptive learning platforms driven by artificial intelligence can personalize content delivery, allowing learners to progress at their own pace and focus on areas needing improvement, thus optimizing educational outcomes. Beyond curriculum development, artificial intelligence also has the potential to enhance existing structures of medical education, from initial training to continuing education.

14.4 Potential of Artificial Intelligence in Existing Health-Care Education

Artificial intelligence has the capacity to revolutionize existing educational structures in health care by making them more responsive, efficient, and learner centered. One of the most significant enhancements lies in the provision of personalized learning pathways. By analyzing individual learner performance, artificial intelligence systems can suggest tailored educational content, ensuring that professionals receive relevant and timely instruction.

Moreover, artificial intelligence can enable immersive clinical simulation environments that mimic complex medical scenarios, allowing learners to practice diagnostics, decision-making, and patient communication in a risk-free setting [21]. A systematic analysis found that artificial intelligence supports all stages of instruction: improved planning by identifying student needs, enhanced implementation through instant feedback, and more efficient assessment with automated tools [22]. These simulations can be enriched through augmented reality and virtual reality, providing a deeply engaging and realistic experience. Administrative tasks can also be streamlined, allowing educators to focus on teaching [23]. Artificial intelligence also supports adaptive instruction, where teaching strategies are dynamically adjusted in real time based on learner feedback and progress. This level of instructional customization promotes higher retention rates and improves overall competency.

14.4.1 Continuous Medical Education with Artificial Intelligence

Continuous medical education traditionally refers to the ongoing professional development activities that health-care professionals engage in to maintain, develop, and increase their knowledge, skills, and professional performance [24]. These traditional activities should expand to encompass emerging digital technology, including telemedicine and artificial intelligence technologies [9, 25, 26]. Integrating continuous medical education seamlessly within the broader framework of medical education ensures that the transition from initial medical training to continuing medical education is smooth and coherent. By embedding continuous medical education principles early, students develop a mindset of continuous learning, preparing them to adapt to new technologies, such as artificial intelligence, throughout their careers. This approach not only facilitates ongoing competency in clinical practice but also instills the agility required to navigate an evolving health-care environment driven by technological innovation.

14.4.2 Artificial Intelligence-Enhanced Continuous Medical Education

This integrated approach aligns medical education with the fast-paced advancements in health care, fostering a culture where ongoing education is not a separate obligation but a natural extension of professional practice [27]. Artificial intelligence-enhanced continuous medical education programs can dynamically identify individual learning gaps and recommend personalized, targeted learning resources, significantly improving educational outcomes. Artificial intelligence-driven analytics provide feedback on learner performance [28], predicting which areas of medical knowledge or clinical skills require attention and allowing proactive remediation. Additionally, integrating artificial intelligence in continuous medical education facilitates real-time updates in response to the latest research findings, regulatory changes, and emerging best practices. This ensures that health-care professionals, whether in training or established practice, remain at the forefront of clinical advancements. By leveraging artificial intelligence, health-care institutions can enhance lifelong learning, reduce barriers to education, and maintain high standards of clinical proficiency across their workforce. Ultimately, this fosters a continuous learning ecosystem where artificial intelligence and health-care education evolve synergistically to meet the needs of modern medical practice [29].

14.5 Potential of Artificial Intelligence in Medical Diagnostic Education

Artificial intelligence's potential in medical diagnostic education is profound. Advanced imaging analysis enables artificial intelligence-powered tools to teach students to interpret complex imaging data, such as computed tomography scans and magnetic resonance imaging, with greater accuracy [30]. Predictive modeling allows learners to explore how artificial intelligence algorithms predict disease progression and outcomes based on historical data. Personalized diagnostic training can be achieved through artificial intelligence systems that adapt to the unique needs of each student, focusing on areas where improvement is needed [31].

Artificial intelligence-based medical interview training enables trainees to practice repeatedly without requiring human simulated patients and supports individual learning [32–34]. This approach also allows trainees to be exposed to challenging scenarios that are difficult to replicate with human simulated patients, such as handling rare or highly sensitive situations, like breaking bad news. Additionally, cultural and linguistic adjustments can be incorporated into the training to better prepare health-care professionals for diverse patient interactions [35]. Our pilot study demonstrated that clinical reasoning using generative artificial intelligence systems in simulated patient scenarios was comparable to that of traditional training stations in Japanese medical interview training. However, some challenges were observed, particularly in communication skills, where artificial intelligence-driven simulations lagged behind traditional stations. This finding highlights the importance of maintaining a balance between innovative artificial intelligence tools and essential human elements of medical training [36].

Despite these advancements, there are challenges associated with overreliance on artificial intelligence-based educational systems. These include the potential for diminished critical thinking, reduced originality in clinical reasoning, and the risk of misinformation if these models are not regularly validated and updated [37–39]. Strategies such as cognitive forcing techniques, which encourage users to consciously question and verify artificial intelligence outputs, have been shown to mitigate these risks [40]. Therefore, medical educators should carefully integrate artificial intelligence-driven education with traditional methods to balance its strengths with the new challenges it presents. By integrating clinical decision support with artificial intelligence-driven diagnostic tools, trainees gain practical experience in combining artificial intelligence insights with clinical judgment, preparing them for real-world scenarios. Artificial intelligence-based medical interview training is also discussed in Chap. 9.

In summary, the integration of artificial intelligence education into health care, particularly in diagnostics, is not just beneficial but essential. By fostering artificial intelligence literacy, developing comprehensive curricula, and leveraging artificial intelligence tools in medical education, we can prepare the next generation of health-care professionals to harness artificial intelligence's full potential responsibly and effectively. As we conclude this discussion on artificial intelligence education, it is imperative to transition our focus towards the horizon of possibilities that artificial intelligence presents. This progression invites us to consider not just the educational frameworks but also the broader implications of artificial intelligence in shaping the future of health-care diagnostics. The final chapter will explore the rapidly evolving landscape of artificial intelligence, highlighting not only the emerging trends and technological breakthroughs but also addressing the strategic challenges that lie ahead. This final chapter aims to provide a comprehensive overview of how innovative artificial intelligence applications are expected to revolutionize diagnostic processes, offering insights into the pathways for sustainable integration and the ethical frameworks necessary for the future of health care.

References

1. Wang C, Chen X, Yu T, Liu Y, Jing Y. Education reform and change driven by digital technology: a bibliometric study from a global perspective. Human Soc Sci Communications. 2024;11(1):256.
2. Doyon P. A review of higher education reform in modern Japan. High Educ. 2001;41:443–70.
3. Bawden D. Origins and concepts of digital literacy. Digital literacies: Concepts, policies and practices, 30 (2008), 17–32. 2008.
4. Eshet Y. Digital literacy: a conceptual framework for survival skills in the digital era. J Educ Multimedia Hypermedia. 2004;13(1):93–106.
5. Tinmaz H, Lee Y-T, Fanea-Ivanovici M, Baber H. A systematic review on digital literacy. Smart Learn Environ. 2022;9(1):21.
6. Long D, Magerko B, editors. What is AI literacy? Competencies and design considerations. Proceedings of the 2020 CHI conference on human factors in computing systems; 2020.
7. Kong S-C, Man-Yin Cheung W, Zhang G. Evaluation of an artificial intelligence literacy course for university students with diverse study backgrounds. Comput Educ Artif Intell. 2021;2:100026.
8. Ng DTK, Leung JKL, Chu SKW, Qiao MS. Conceptualizing AI literacy: an exploratory review. Comput Educ Artif Intell. 2021;2:100041.
9. Laupichler MC, Aster A, Schirch J, Raupach T. Artificial intelligence literacy in higher and adult education: a scoping literature review. Comput Educ Artif Intell. 2022;3:100101.
10. Li H, Klabjan D. Reverse Prompt Engineering arXiv preprint arXiv:241106729. 2024.
11. Sampson JR. Adaptation in natural and artificial systems (John H. Holland). SIAM Rev. 1976;18(3):529–2.
12. Gazquez-Garcia J, Sánchez-Bocanegra CL, Sevillano JL. AI in the health sector: systematic review of key skills for future health professionals. JMIR Med Educ. 2025;11:e58161.

13. Yin J, Ngiam KY, Teo HH. Role of artificial intelligence applications in real-life clinical practice: systematic review. J Med Internet Res. 2021;23(4):e25759.
14. McCoy LG, Nagaraj S, Morgado F, Harish V, Das S, Celi LA. What do medical students actually need to know about artificial intelligence? NPJ Digit Med. 2020;3(1):86.
15. Liaw W, Kueper JK, Lin S, Bazemore A, Kakadiaris I. Competencies for the use of artificial intelligence in primary care. Annals Family Med. 2022;20(6):559–63.
16. Çalışkan SA, Demir K, Karaca O. Artificial intelligence in medical education curriculum: an e-Delphi study for competencies. PLoS One. 2022;17(7):e0271872.
17. Marwaha JS, Landman AB, Brat GA, Dunn T, Gordon WJ. Deploying digital health tools within large, complex health systems: key considerations for adoption and implementation. NPJ Digit Med. 2022;5(1):13.
18. Tejani AS. Identifying and addressing barriers to an artificial intelligence curriculum. J Am Coll Radiol. 2021;18(4):605–7.
19. Grunhut J, Marques O, Wyatt ATM. Needs, challenges, and applications of artificial intelligence in medical education curriculum. JMIR Med Educ. 2022;8(2):e35587.
20. Longhini J, Rossettini G, Palese A. Digital health competencies among health care professionals: systematic review. J Med Internet Res. 2022;24(8):e36414.
21. Lampropoulos G. Combining artificial intelligence with augmented reality and virtual reality in education: current trends and future perspectives. Multimodal Technol Interact. 2025;9(2):11.
22. Celik I, Dindar M, Muukkonen H, Järvelä S. The promises and challenges of artificial intelligence for teachers: a systematic review of research. TechTrends. 2022;66(4):616–30.
23. Chen L, Chen P, Lin Z. Artificial intelligence in education: a review. IEEE Access. 2020;8:75264–78.
24. Davis DA, Thomson MA, Oxman AD, Haynes RB. Changing physician performance: a systematic review of the effect of continuing medical education strategies. JAMA. 1995;274(9):700–5.
25. Waseh S, Dicker AP. Telemedicine training in undergraduate medical education: mixed-methods review. JMIR Med Educ. 2019;5(1):e12515-e.
26. O'Shea J, Berger R, Samra C, Van Durme D. Telemedicine in education: bridging the gap. Educ Health (Abingdon). 2015;28(1):64–7.
27. Cooper A, Rodman A. AI and medical education — a 21st-century Pandora's box. N Engl J Med. 2023;389(5):385–7.
28. Huang C-J, Wang Y-W, Huang T-H, Chen Y-C, Chen H-M, Chang S-C. Performance evaluation of an online argumentation learning assistance agent. Comput Educ. 2011;57(1):1270–80.
29. Li R, Wu T. Evolution of artificial intelligence in medical education from 2000 to 2024: bibliometric analysis. Interact J Med Res. 2025;14:e63775.
30. Li MD, Little BP. Appropriate reliance on artificial intelligence in radiology education. J Am Coll Radiol. 2023;20(11):1126–30.
31. Strielkowski W, Grebennikova V, Lisovskiy A, Rakhimova G, Vasileva T. AI-driven adaptive learning for sustainable educational transformation. Sustain Dev. 2025;33(2):1921–47.
32. White CB, Wendling A, Lampotang S, Lizdas D, Cordar A, Lok B. The role for virtual patients in the future of medical education. Acad Med. 2017;92(1):10–9.
33. Potter L, Jefferies C. Enhancing communication and clinical reasoning in medical education: building virtual patients with generative AI. Future Healthcare J. 2024;11:100043.
34. Yamamoto A, Koda M, Ogawa H, Miyoshi T, Maeda Y, Otsuka F, et al. Enhancing medical interview skills through AI-simulated patient interactions: nonrandomized controlled trial. JMIR Med Educ. 2024;10:e58753.
35. Schouten BC, Meeuwesen L. Cultural differences in medical communication: a review of the literature. Patient Educ Couns. 2006;64(1):21–34.
36. Hirosawa T, Yokose M, Sakamoto T, Harada Y, Tokumasu K, Mizuta K, et al. Utility of generative artificial intelligence for Japanese medical interview training: randomized crossover pilot study. JMIR Med Educ. 2025;11:e77332.
37. Lucas HC, Upperman JS, Robinson JR. A systematic review of large language models and their implications in medical education. Med Educ. 2024;58:1276.

38. Passi S, Vorvoreanu M. Overreliance on AI Literature Review 2022. Available from: https://www.microsoft.com/en-us/research/uploads/prod/2022/06/Aether-Overreliance-on-AI-Review-Final-6.21.22.pdf
39. Bair H, Norden J. Large language models and their implications on medical education. Acad Med. 2023;98(8):869.
40. Buçinca Z, Malaya MB, Gajos KZ. To trust or to think: cognitive forcing functions can reduce overreliance on AI in AI-assisted decision-making. Proc ACM Human Comput Interact. 2021;5(CSCW1):1–21.

15 The Future Direction of AI in Diagnostics

Abstract

This last chapter summarizes the previous chapters and explores the future direction of artificial intelligence in medical diagnostics. The chapter examines the evolution of artificial intelligence technology, addressing breakthroughs such as quantum computing, neuromorphic computing, and biocomputing, alongside the transformative impact of artificial intelligence-enhanced health care. The discussion will explore hyper-scale, specialized, and edge artificial intelligence. These systems offer integrated electronic health records and public health advancements. Moreover, it highlights the collaborative potential of hybrid intelligence, the synergy of human, and the artificial intelligence capabilities, in shaping the future of medical diagnostics and transforming patient care.

Keywords

Hybrid intelligence · Quantum computing · Edge computing · Telemedicine · Personalized medicine · Public health

15.1 The Future Direction of Artificial Intelligence

15.1.1 Hyper-Scale Artificial Intelligence, Specialized Artificial Intelligence, and Edge Artificial Intelligence

Technology giants, such as Google, Amazon, Meta, Microsoft, and Apple, are increasingly investing in hyper-scale artificial intelligence systems. Hyper-scale artificial intelligence refers to an expansive and high-performance system designed to manage vast datasets and extensive computations across a wide variety of applications. These artificial intelligence systems offer integrated and comprehensive solutions capable of addressing multiple complex tasks. Concurrently, there is

T. Hirosawa, *Artificial Intelligence in Medical Diagnostics*,
https://doi.org/10.1007/978-981-95-4338-0_15

growing enthusiasm for artificial general intelligence, an ambitious area of artificial intelligence research aiming to create systems with human-like cognitive abilities, enabling them to learn, reason, and perform diverse tasks without being explicitly programmed for each function [1]. While artificial general intelligence is still in early development, it represents the frontier of artificial intelligence development, pushing the boundaries of what artificial intelligence can achieve across multiple domains, including health care.

In contrast, specialized artificial intelligence systems are described as small-scale artificial intelligence. They are precision-oriented technologies designed to address distinct domain-specific challenges, including medical or diagnostic contexts within specific health-care domains or specialties. These systems have distinct advantages, such as their ability to operate as stand-alone tools without the need for extensive infrastructure [2]. This independence significantly enhances their practicability and utility, especially in resource-limited settings where advanced technological infrastructure is unavailable or financially prohibitive. Specialized artificial intelligence tools often operate on localized hardware, reducing reliance on cloud-based systems and ensuring critical health-care operations remain uninterrupted and efficient. Moreover, the lower development and deployment costs make these systems a cost-effective solution, enabling wider adoption and improved health-care delivery in underserved areas. The stand-alone nature is also beneficial for inputting sensitive patient information, ensuring privacy and reducing dependency on external networks or centralized data systems.

Edge artificial intelligence, closely associated with specialized artificial intelligence, incorporates principles of edge computing. Edge computing is a distributed computing framework that brings computation and data storage closer to the location where it is needed [3]. For example, edge computing applications like a fog computing-based Fall Monitoring System for Stroke Mitigation demonstrate how small artificial intelligence can address critical health-care issues by monitoring stroke risks and reducing severity [4, 5]. Other systems, such as eWALL for managing chronic obstructive pulmonary disease and mild dementia, highlight how distributed artificial intelligence architectures can process sensitive patient information locally, reducing communication overhead while maintaining real-time functionality [6].

The separation between hyper-scale artificial intelligence and specialized or edge artificial intelligence reflects essential strategic considerations within medical diagnostics technology development. Hyper-scale artificial intelligence's strength lies in handling complex, large-scale clinical data analysis and integrating various health-care services, making it ideal for comprehensive health-care systems. Conversely, specialized and edge artificial intelligence offer targeted, cost-effective solutions tailored to specific diagnostic needs or health-care contexts, highlighting their critical role in health-care accessibility. This dichotomy represents a vital future direction, as both hyper-scale and specialized artificial intelligence contribute to advancements in their respective scopes [7], as shown in Table 15.1.

Table 15.1 Comparison between hyper-scale and specialized artificial intelligence (AI)

Aspect	Hyper-scale AI	Specialized AI
Definition	Expansive systems for broad applications	Targeted tools for specific challenges
Scope	General intelligence with human-like cognitive abilities across domains	Narrow focus on discrete tasks such as health care or diagnostics
Infrastructure	Extensive computational and infrastructural requirements	Stand-alone tools leveraging edge computing
Applications	Broad applications across multiple domains	Specific health care uses, e.g., stroke monitoring, chronic disease management, eWALL
Advantages	Comprehensive, integrated solutions pushing AI boundaries	Lower cost, accessible, adaptable, ensuring data privacy
Data processing	Centralized or large-scale processing	Localized processing reducing communication overhead
Cost	High development and deployment costs	Lower development and deployment costs
Future direction	Advancements across diverse fields	Efficiency and accessibility in specialized domains

15.1.2 Integration with Other Systems, Including Electronic Health Records

The integration of artificial intelligence into electronic health records and other health-care systems is emerging as a cornerstone for the future of artificial intelligence in diagnostics. By incorporating artificial intelligence technologies into these systems, health-care professionals can ensure seamless data sharing and analysis, fostering more effective and timely decision-making. This integration also enables the personalization of medical treatments, allowing practitioners to tailor interventions to individual patient needs based on comprehensive data insights [8].

15.1.3 Technological Breakthrough

Current developments in artificial intelligence face several technological bottlenecks, including limitations in computing hardware capabilities, energy efficiency, dataset availability, and operational costs. The prevalent artificial intelligence systems rely on machine learning models that require large and high-quality datasets for effective training to accurately identify patterns and generate meaningful insights. However, acquiring extensive and high-quality medical data remains a significant challenge due to privacy concerns, restricted access, and the heterogeneous nature of medical records across institutions. This challenge limits the efficacy and applicability of traditional machine learning models in real-world medical diagnostics.

To resolve these dataset and computational constraints, researchers are exploring alternative approaches, such as chain-of-thought reasoning models. These models adopt a structured reasoning process, enabling artificial intelligence systems to perform logical analyses rather than relying solely on pattern recognition. This methodological shift not only enhances model interpretability but also provides health-care professionals with greater confidence and transparency in artificial intelligence-generated diagnostic recommendations, thereby significantly improving clinical relevance and trustworthiness [9, 10].

Quantum computing technology represents another significant advancement in addressing the limitations within traditional computational paradigms [11]. By exploring quantum mechanical phenomena, quantum computing can potentially solve highly complex computational problems at speeds unattainable by classical computing methods. Consequently, it opens new avenues for enhancing the capabilities of artificial intelligence, particularly in complex diagnostics tasks, including the analysis of large-scale genomic data or complex biological systems. Despite its potential, quantum computing still faces substantial technical hurdles, such as error correction, quantum bit (qubit) stability, coherence, connectivity, and scalability [12].

Another critical breakthrough lies in neuromorphic computing, which emulates the neural structure of the human brain to improve energy efficiency and processing capabilities. This approach could significantly enhance artificial intelligence's capacity to perform real-time tasks with minimal power consumption. In addition, advancements in photonic computing—leveraging light instead of electrons for data transmission—hold promise for ultrafast artificial intelligence systems with reduced latency [13].

Emerging materials science innovations, such as the development of memristors, also represent a breakthrough in artificial intelligence technology. Memristors, which can retain memory without power, enable faster and more efficient data storage and processing. This advancement could revolutionize edge computing applications by allowing devices to process data locally with enhanced speed and energy efficiency [14, 15].

Furthermore, biocomputing, which uses biological molecules like DNA and proteins to perform computations, is another frontier [16]. Biocomputing holds the potential for unprecedented processing power with extremely low energy requirements. Its potential to enable highly personalized diagnostics and treatment planning through complex biological computations positions biocomputing as a revolutionary development, particularly in precision medicine.

These multiple breakthroughs—ranging from quantum and neuromorphic computing to photonic systems, memristor technology, and biocomputing—hold transformative potential to overcome current artificial intelligence limitations. Collectively, these advancements could lead to a new era of highly capable, efficient, and clinically impactful artificial intelligence solutions, thereby significantly advancing the field of medical diagnostics and enhancing overall health care outcomes. Alongside these technological breakthroughs, it is the broader integration of artificial intelligence into health systems that will truly define its future trajectory.

15.2 The Future Direction of Health Care with Artificial Intelligence

15.2.1 Public Health

Artificial intelligence offers transformative potential in addressing public health challenges, particularly mitigating health inequities. Artificial intelligence-powered solutions can provide scalable diagnostic and treatment options for underserved communities, ensuring that health-care resources reach populations with limited access [17]. Furthermore, advanced artificial intelligence algorithms excel at identifying trends within large datasets, enabling the prediction and prevention of public health crises. Through these capabilities, artificial intelligence fosters equitable and proactive approaches to health care [18].

15.2.2 Integration with Telemedicine

The integration of artificial intelligence with telemedicine platforms represents a pivotal advancement in health-care delivery. By merging artificial intelligence diagnostic tools with telehealth services, providers can offer real-time consultations and assessments regardless of geographical barriers. This integration not only improves the accessibility of care for remote or underserved populations but also enhances diagnostic accuracy through artificial intelligence-driven insights. As telemedicine becomes an integral part of modern health care, artificial intelligence ensures that these services are both efficient and effective [19].

15.2.3 Integration with Research

Current advancements in artificial intelligence research have demonstrated remarkable integration of tools such as AlphaFold, which predicts protein structures with unprecedented accuracy [20, 21]. This breakthrough has revolutionized the field of molecular biology by providing insights into protein folding mechanisms, aiding drug discovery, and enhancing our understanding of various diseases. Building on these advancements, the future of artificial intelligence research is poised to expand into more complex domains, where multidisciplinary approaches combine computational power with experimental validation to address critical challenges in medicine and beyond.

Artificial intelligence is revolutionizing the field of medical research by enabling real-time systematic reviews, living systematic reviews, and continuous analysis of emerging data [22–24]. This capability allows researchers to stay updated with the latest findings and incorporate them into clinical practices. By automating the synthesis of vast volumes of research data, artificial intelligence accelerates innovation and ensures that medical advancements are both timely and impactful.

In addition to real-time reviews, artificial intelligence supports diagnostic research by generating evaluations for differential diagnosis lists, including the identification of the most likely final diagnosis [25]. This capability enables health-care professionals to systematically compare and prioritize potential conditions, streamlining the decision-making process and enhancing the overall accuracy and reliability of diagnostic outcomes.

15.2.4 The Future Direction of Medical Diagnostics

Research demonstrates that artificial intelligence systems can enhance human performance, particularly those with less experience. For instance, studies have shown that artificial intelligence tools provide substantial support to beginners, helping them achieve outcomes comparable to skilled workers. From a nonmedical study, this aligns with findings of approximately 5000 customer support agents, which revealed that access to generative artificial intelligence tools increased productivity by 14% on average. Low-skilled workers experienced a 34% improvement, while the impact on experienced workers was minimal [26]. The study suggested that artificial intelligence disseminates best practices of skilled workers, aiding newer individuals to accelerate their performance.

In medical diagnostics, these principles are particularly applicable in areas such as radiology and pathology, where pattern recognition is an essential component for experts [27, 28]. These fields require precise identification of subtle patterns based on rich clinical experience. These results are critical for accurate diagnosis and treatment planning where artificial intelligence-powered tools assist in identifying subtle patterns that may elude human observation. For instance, artificial intelligence algorithms trained on large datasets of medical images can detect early signs of diseases such as cancer with remarkable precision, supporting less experienced radiologists in making accurate diagnoses. Furthermore, these tools not only enhance diagnostic accuracy but also improve efficiency by significantly reducing the time required for analysis. In clinical settings, artificial intelligence can facilitate triage by prioritizing cases requiring immediate attention, allowing health-care professionals to allocate resources more effectively. These advancements emphasize the transformative potential of artificial intelligence in elevating diagnostic practices across the medical field. These insights indicate that the collaboration between human expertise and artificial intelligence not only augments diagnostic accuracy but also fosters learning and confidence among emerging professionals [29].

15.3 The Future Direction of Intelligence

15.3.1 Hybrid Intelligence

The concept of hybrid intelligence, sometimes referred to as hybrid-augmented intelligence [30], highlights the symbiotic relationship between artificial intelligence systems and human intelligence, including health-care professionals and patients in medical contexts. Artificial intelligence learns from datasets created by humans, ensuring that its outputs are based on human knowledge and expertise. We must also adopt the stance of absorbing all outputs from artificial intelligence, critically analyzing them to refine and enhance future processes. This reciprocal interaction strengthens the synergy between humans and artificial intelligence. By leveraging the complementary strengths of both, hybrid intelligence facilitates diagnostic decisions that are not only accurate but also contextually nuanced. This approach ensures that artificial intelligence systems function as supportive tools rather than replacements, enriching the diagnostic process [31, 32].

For example, a collaborative workflow can be envisioned where users understand artificial intelligence mechanisms well enough to input data of adequate quality and quantity into the system. Artificial intelligence then generates outputs, which the user critically evaluates, refines, and uses to improve the next input. This iterative process, resembling a circulation, combines the strengths of human critical thinking and artificial intelligence's analytical power, leading to continuous improvement and enhanced diagnostic precision. This concept is illustrated in Fig. 15.1.

In Fig. 15.2, the progression of intelligence in diagnostics is depicted, transitioning from traditional reliance on human intelligence alone to the current coexistence of human and artificial intelligence. The future envisions a hybrid intelligence model where human and artificial intelligence systems mutually influence and enhance each other's capabilities. Human intelligence, shaped by insights and patterns identified by artificial intelligence, grows more informed and precise, while artificial intelligence, informed by human expertise, becomes more contextually adaptive and reliable. This progression of intelligence would improve both human and artificial intelligence, fostering a mutually beneficial evolution in their capabilities [33, 34].

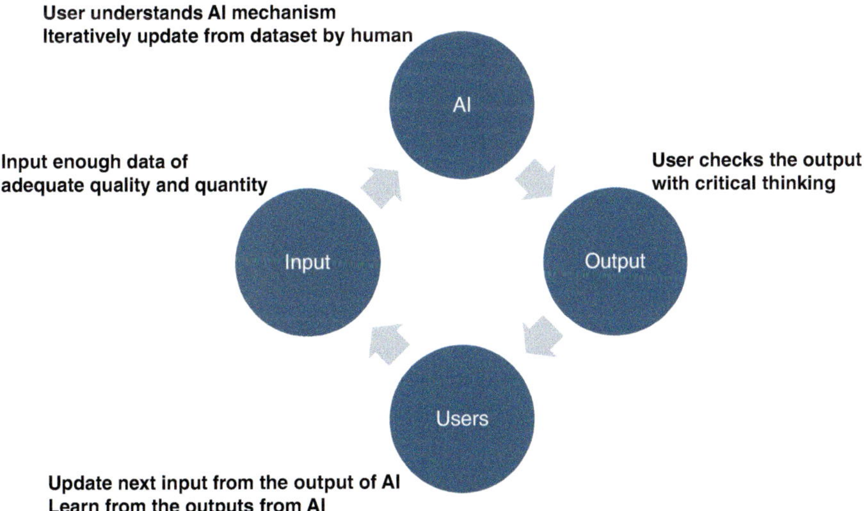

Fig. 15.1 Concept of collaboration with users and artificial intelligence (AI)

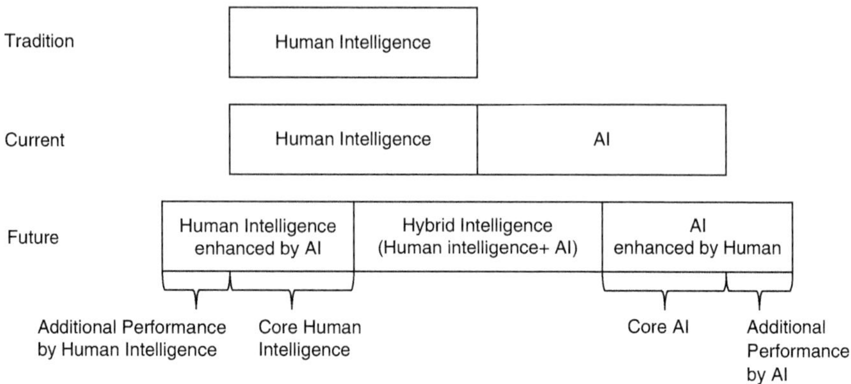

Fig. 15.2 Concept of collaboration with human intelligence and artificial intelligence (AI)

15.3.2 Collaboration with Human and Artificial Intelligence in Medicine

The future of medical diagnostics is characterized by deep collaboration between health-care professionals and artificial intelligence technologies. These partnerships enhance the reliability, precision, and accessibility of diagnostics, resulting in improved patient care [35].

Early prediction is one area where artificial intelligence excels, enabling health-care professionals to identify potential health issues well before symptoms manifest, thereby allowing for timely interventions. For instance, artificial intelligence can detect early signs of atrial fibrillation by analyzing subtle patterns in heart rate variability before irregularly irregular rhythms occur [36]. This early detection enables timely medical interventions, potentially preventing complications such as stroke and heart failure [37].

Additionally, artificial intelligence facilitates personalized medicine by analyzing a patient's unique genetic, environmental, and lifestyle factors to develop tailored treatment plans. Physical artificial intelligence [38]—such as robotics integrated with diagnostic and therapeutic systems—also contributes by automating repetitive tasks and performing precision-guided procedures, particularly in imaging-guided interventions. By combining the analytical capabilities of artificial intelligence with the contextual understanding of human professionals, this collaborative model represents a balanced and effective approach to medical diagnostics.

Looking ahead, artificial intelligence could also drive advancements in integrating real-time patient monitoring systems with diagnostic platforms, offering a seamless and proactive approach to patient care.

15.4 Conclusion

In conclusion, artificial intelligence has significant potential to improve human performance, particularly in medicine and, most importantly, medical diagnostics. These technologies have demonstrated considerable promise in increasing diagnostic precision, facilitating early disease prediction, and enabling highly personalized interventions. Consequently, artificial intelligence is poised to revolutionize health-care delivery, making it more effective, efficient, and responsive to individual patient needs. To realize this vision, we must carefully and rigorously develop, evaluate, and integrate these digital technologies into existing medical workflows, ensuring they amplify benefits while minimizing potential risks.

The rapid advancements in artificial intelligence present us with the opportunity and challenge to redefine our very understanding of intelligence. They compel us to deeply reconsider how digital technologies can reshape not only diagnostic processes but also broader health-care experiences. For health-care professionals, this transformative shift necessitates rethinking traditional clinical workflows, diagnostic methodologies, and clinical decision-making processes to effectively integrate artificial intelligence tools. For patients, the rise of artificial intelligence in health care prompts critical discussions around issues of trust, data privacy, and the balance between technology-driven insights and human empathy in care delivery.

Artificial intelligence also provokes philosophical reflections on the essence of human-specific intelligence, especially heuristic reasoning and intuition, which traditionally underpin clinical decision-making. Generative artificial intelligence challenges our notions of creativity, originality, and innovation within human-machine collaborations, leading us to reconsider the distinctions and overlaps between human and artificial creativity. Similarly, neural networks, by mimicking the brain's architecture, invite us to explore more deeply into human cognition. Likewise, large language models prompt us to reexamine the profundity of language as a distinctly human tool and its evolving role within communication including in health-care contexts.

Through this book, we have highlighted that successfully navigating these profound technical shifts demands a collaborative effort among diverse stakeholders. Scientists, health-care professionals, policymakers, patients, their families, and the broader society all play essential roles in shaping the responsible adoption of artificial intelligence. By fostering meaningful collaborations between humans and artificial intelligence, we can harness the full potential of these tools to not only improve specific domains like health care but also to drive broader societal transformation.

I hope this book opens readers' eyes to the importance of collaboration and bridging the gap between artificial intelligence and medicine to shape a better future. Only through thoughtful collaboration and mutual understanding can we fully harness artificial intelligence's transformative potential to address pressing global health-care challenges. Collectively, our shared goal must be to cultivate a future where human and artificial intelligence evolve synergistically, improving outcomes, enhancing human experiences, and fostering continuous growth for the betterment of all.

References

1. Fahad M, Basri T, Hamza MA, Faisal S, Akbar A, Haider U, et al. The benefits and risks of Artificial General Intelligence (AGI). In: El Hajjami S, Kaushik K, Khan IU, editors. Artificial General Intelligence (AGI) security: smart applications and sustainable technologies. Singapore: Springer; 2025. p. 27–52.
2. Singh R, Gill SS. Edge AI: a survey. Internet Things Cyber-Phys Syst. 2023;3:71–92.
3. Khan WZ, Ahmed E, Hakak S, Yaqoob I, Ahmed A. Edge computing: a survey. Futur Gener Comput Syst. 2019;97:219–35.
4. Craciunescu R, Mihovska A, Mihaylov M, Kyriazakos S, Prasad R, Halunga S, editors. Implementation of Fog computing for reliable E-health applications. 2015 49th Asilomar conference on signals, systems and computers. IEEE; 2015.
5. Cao K, Liu Y, Meng G, Sun Q. An overview on edge computing research. IEEE Access. 2020;8:85714–28.
6. Fratu O, Pena C, Craciunescu R, Halunga S, editors. Fog computing system for monitoring Mild Dementia and COPD patients-Romanian case study.. 2015 12th international conference on telecommunication in modern satellite, cable and broadcasting services (TELSIKS); 2015: IEEE.
7. Wang YC, Xue J, Wei C, Kuo CCJ. An overview on generative AI at scale with edge–cloud computing. IEEE Open J Commun Soc. 2023;4:2952–71.
8. Knevel R, Liao KP. From real-world electronic health record data to real-world results using artificial intelligence. Ann Rheum Dis. 2023;82(3):306–11.
9. Wei J, Wang X, Schuurmans D, Bosma M, Xia F, Chi E, et al. Chain-of-thought prompting elicits reasoning in large language models. Adv Neural Inf Proces Syst. 2022;35:24824–37.
10. Yu F, Zhang H, Tiwari P, Wang B. Natural language reasoning, a survey. ACM Comput Surv. 2024;56(12):Article 304.
11. Gyongyosi L, Imre S. A survey on quantum computing technology. Comput Sci Rev. 2019;31:51–71.
12. Gill SS, Kumar A, Singh H, Singh M, Kaur K, Usman M, et al. Quantum computing: a taxonomy, systematic review and future directions. Softw Pract Exp. 2022;52(1):66–114.
13. Kudithipudi D, Schuman C, Vineyard CM, Pandit T, Merkel C, Kubendran R, et al. Neuromorphic computing at scale. Nature. 2025;637(8047):801–12.
14. Youngblood N, Ríos Ocampo CA, Pernice WHP, Bhaskaran H. Integrated optical memristors. Nat Photonics. 2023;17(7):561–72.
15. Huang Y, Ando T, Sebastian A, Chang M-F, Yang JJ, Xia Q. Memristor-based hardware accelerators for artificial intelligence. Nat Rev Electr Eng. 2024;1(5):286–99.
16. Qiu X, Zhu L, Wang H, Xie M. Biocomputing at the crossroad between emulating artificial intelligence and cellular supremacy. Curr Opin Biotechnol. 2025;92:103264.
17. Dangi RR, Sharma A, Vageriya V. Transforming healthcare in low-resource settings with artificial intelligence: recent developments and outcomes. Public Health Nurs. 2025;42(2):1017–30.
18. Schwalbe N, Wahl B. Artificial intelligence and the future of global health. Lancet. 2020;395(10236):1579–86.
19. Sharma S, Rawal R, Shah D. Addressing the challenges of AI-based telemedicine: best practices and lessons learned. J Educ Health Promot. 2023;12:338.
20. Abramson J, Adler J, Dunger J, Evans R, Green T, Pritzel A, et al. Accurate structure prediction of biomolecular interactions with AlphaFold 3. Nature. 2024;630(8016):493–500.

21. Li B, Gilbert S. Artificial intelligence awarded two Nobel prizes for innovations that will shape the future of medicine. NPJ Digit Med. 2024;7(1):336.
22. Marshall IJ, Trikalinos TA, Soboczenski F, Yun HS, Kell G, Marshall R, et al. In a pilot study, automated real-time systematic review updates were feasible, accurate, and work-saving. J Clin Epidemiol. 2023;153:26–33.
23. Schmidt L, Sinyor M, Webb RT, Marshall C, Knipe D, Eyles EC, et al. A narrative review of recent tools and innovations toward automating living systematic reviews and evidence syntheses. Z Evid Fortbild Qual Gesundhwes. 2023;181:65–75.
24. Breuer C, Meerpohl JJ, Siemens W. From standard systematic reviews to living systematic reviews. Z Evid Fortbild Qual Gesundhwes. 2023;176:76–81.
25. Hirosawa T, Harada Y, Mizuta K, Sakamoto T, Tokumasu K, Shimizu T. Evaluating ChatGPT-4's accuracy in identifying final diagnoses within differential diagnoses compared with those of physicians: experimental study for diagnostic cases. JMIR Form Res. 2024;8:e59267.
26. Brynjolfsson E, Li D, Raymond LR. Generative AI at work. National Bureau of Economic Research; 2023.
27. Kelly BS, Judge C, Bollard SM, Clifford SM, Healy GM, Aziz A, et al. Radiology artificial intelligence: a systematic review and evaluation of methods (RAISE). Eur Radiol. 2022;32(11):7998–8007.
28. Shafi S, Parwani AV. Artificial intelligence in diagnostic pathology. Diagn Pathol. 2023;18(1):109.
29. Sahu M, Gupta R, Ambasta RK, Kumar P. Chapter three – Artificial intelligence and machine learning in precision medicine: a paradigm shift in big data analysis. In: Teplow DB, editor. Progress in molecular biology and translational science, vol. 190. Academic; 2022. p. 57–100.
30. Zheng N-n, Liu Z-y, Ren P-j, Ma Y-q, Chen S-t, Yu S-y, et al. Hybrid-augmented intelligence: collaboration and cognition. Front Inf Technol Electron Eng. 2017;18(2):153–79.
31. Hirosawa T, Suzuki T, Shiraishi T, Hayashi A, Fujii Y, Harada T, et al. Adapting artificial intelligence concepts to enhance clinical decision-making: a hybrid intelligence framework. Int J Gen Med. 2024;17:5417–22.
32. Nazar M, Alam MM, Yafi E, Su'ud MM. A systematic review of human–computer interaction and explainable artificial intelligence in healthcare with artificial intelligence techniques. IEEE Access. 2021;9:153316–48.
33. Jarrahi MH, Lutz C, Newlands G. Artificial intelligence, human intelligence and hybrid intelligence based on mutual augmentation. Big Data Soc. 2022;9(2):20539517221142824.
34. Deng C, Ji X, Rainey C, Zhang J, Lu W. Integrating machine learning with human knowledge. iScience. 2020;23(11):101656.
35. Bellini V, Badino M, Maffezzoni M, Bezzi F, Bignami E. Evolution of hybrid intelligence and its application in evidence-based medicine: a review. Med Sci Monit. 2023;29:e939366.
36. Wang Y-C, Xu X, Hajra A, Apple S, Kharawala A, Duarte G, et al. Current advancement in diagnosing atrial fibrillation by utilizing wearable devices and artificial intelligence: a review study. Diagnostics. 2022;12(3):689.
37. Kirchhof P. The future of atrial fibrillation management: integrated care and stratified therapy. Lancet. 2017;390(10105):1873–87.
38. Miriyev A, Kovač M. Skills for physical artificial intelligence. Nat Mach Intell. 2020;2(11):658–60.